Gerontological Nursing Review

A Self-Instructional Text

Gerontological Nursing Review

A Self-Instructional Text

Charlotte Eliopoulos, R.N.C., M.P.H.

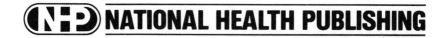 NATIONAL HEALTH PUBLISHING

Printed in the United States of America
First Printing
ISBN:0-932500-76-5
LC: 87-62120

To my grandparents

Contents

Practice Issues 82

Service Delivery *82* Legal Aspects *85*
Reimbursement *89* Assuring Quality *90* Research *92*
Gerontological Nursing as a Specialty *93*

Preface

Increasing numbers of nurses are discovering the challenges and rewards of working with older adults in a wide range of care settings. Often, nurses discover that gerontological nursing is much more complex than they ever imagined. The different norms and manifestations of illness, the multiple losses, psychosocial dynamics, ethical dilemmas, service networks, and constantly changing benefit programs of the elderly population make the nursing care of other age groups seem simple by comparison.

Although gerontological nursing is a unique and complex specialty, few nurses have received specialized preparation in this area. Only recently have nursing schools included courses and graduate programs in gerontological nursing. The majority of nurses working with older adults have not had the benefit of such academic preparation; they have had to gain their knowledge "the hard way" by attending whatever continuing education programs they could find and by reading independently. This book strives to make the burden on these nurses a little lighter.

Gerontological Nursing Review is a short, practical text aimed to help nurses:

- assess their existing knowledge and skills in gerontological nursing
- gain a knowledge base in gerontological nursing
- prepare for the Gerontological Nursing Certification Examination given by the American Nurses' Association.

The text begins with a 100-item, multiple-choice examination similar to the ANA Certification test. To help sharpen test-taking skills, hints are provided in the back of the book. The reader should take the test in Part I first and then proceed to the test review in Part II, which will analyze the correct answer. After reading the text, the reader should take the exam again to determine which subjects require more intense study. The bibliography lists readings related to specific topics covered in the test so that readers can seek additional resources on those subjects they find most difficult.

It is hoped that this review will aid nurses in identifying the scope and complexity of gerontological nursing and serve as a stimulus for further learning activities.

For information related to exact dates and locations of the certification exam, contact the American Nurses' Association, 2420 Pershing Road, Kansas City, Missouri, 64108.

Acknowledgments

I am deeply indebted to the many nurses who have attended my Gerontological Nursing Review workshops over the years, aided me in refining content, and encouraged me to publish this material so that an additional resource would be available to assist nurses in independent review.

Also, I am grateful to Terry Altimont and other Rynd Communications staff for their valuable assistance and support throughout the book's development.

About the Author

Charlotte Eliopoulos, RNC, MPH, has demonstrated leadership in gerontological nursing as an author, lecturer, and initiator of new roles. At the Johns Hopkins Hospital during the 1970s, she developed a gerontological clinical specialist position considered to be the first such position in an acute care setting in the U.S. She then went on to serve as the first state-level specialist in gerontological nursing for the Maryland Department of Health. Later, she became Vice President for Nursing at Levindale Geriatric Center and Hospital where she was involved in the management of the nursing home units, chronic hospital, geriatric day care program, and other services. She now is in private practice, writing and providing consultation and education for geriatric care providers.

Ms. Eliopoulos holds a diploma in nursing from Sinai Hospital in Baltimore and bachelor's and master's degrees from the Johns Hopkins University. She has been certified in gerontological nursing for over 10 years and has served on the ANA's Gerontological Nursing Certification Board.

In addition to numerous articles, Ms. Eliopoulos has published several other texts including *Gerontological Nursing, Health Assessment of the Older Adult,* and *Nursing Administration of Long Term Care.*

PART I:

Gerontological Nursing Test

Gerontological Nursing Review
Test Questions

1. *Which statement best describes the older population in the United States?*

    a. It is predominantly male.
    b. It is comprised of greater numbers of "old-old."
    c. It is becoming a smaller percentage of the total population.
    d. It is enjoying a longer lifespan than previous generations.

2. *You relocate to a new state and are interested in working with older adults in the community. In surveying available services, you discover that most geriatric programs are located in urban areas. The most likely reason for this is:*

    a. City governments have placed higher priority on the elderly than county governments
    b. Rural and suburban elderly are less responsive to formal services than urban elderly
    c. Families in rural and suburban areas provide more services to older relatives than those in urban areas
    d. The largest number of elderly are found in urban areas

3. *Which situation is most typical of the living arrangements of most older adults?*

    a. An older man living in a rooming house alone
    b. Two sisters sharing an apartment
    c. A married couple living in the community
    d. A widow living in her children's home

4. *A group of neighbors ranging in ages from 64 to 76 meet for lunch weekly. All of the women are widowed. Which statement best describes their widowhood?*

    a. They are atypical of most older women.

    b. They represent the reality for most older women.
    c. Few women in their age group are widowed.
    d. They are outnumbered by widowers at that age.

5. *You are leading a discussion group for middle-aged persons who wish to learn more about their elderly parents. As the participants share their own family experiences, which statement would you recognize as describing an unusual situation?*
    a. "My parents and I live within a half-hour of each other, and we all prefer that arrangement."
    b. "My mother and father had a rocky marriage for years, but now they seem to have calmed down and get along better."
    c. "My parents and I are in touch at least once a week."
    d. "My mother and her sister used to be close, but they now have drifted apart."

6. *As compared with white elderly, older blacks:*
    a. Do not live as long, but have strong family ties
    b. Are poorer, although healthier
    c. Have a male life expectancy that exceeds that of females
    d. Have a higher rate of institutionalization

7. *You are a new public health nurse on an American Indian reservation. In establishing priorities for the health screening of this group, the high-risk problem that you would be most interested in addressing is:*
    a. Violence
    b. Tuberculosis
    c. Alcoholism
    d. Pancreatic cancer

8. *Which is true regarding older Orientals in the U.S.?*
    a. They are held in high esteem by their families.
    b. Most have settled in New York.
    c. They have experienced very little prejudice.
    d. There is a higher female:male ratio among older Chinese than among the non-Oriental elderly.

9. *As a new public health nurse, you find that there are many Hispanics in your community, and you wish to address their unique interests and needs. Which of the following actions would be most appropriate for this group?*

    a. Helping them establish a nursing home in their community
    b. Developing caregiver education and support
    c. Suspending home visits from sundown Friday to sunrise Saturday
    d. Utilizing lay healers

10. *What is the primary source of income for most older individuals?*

    a. Employment earnings
    b. Private pensions
    c. Social Security
    d. Investment income

11. *Regarding the financial status of the elderly, which is a true statement?*

    a. Older women possess more wealth and income than their male counterparts.
    b. The percentage of elderly in the poverty level has been steadily declining.
    c. There is no significant difference between the income of black and white elderly.
    d. A majority of retirees have incomes from private pension plans.

12. *Which statement would you know to be a fact regarding the rate of illness in old age?*

    a. Chronic illness occurs at four times the rate as in younger years, while acute illness occurs at one-half the rate.
    b. Acute and chronic illness occur at the same rate.
    c. The rate of acute illness begins to exceed the rate of chronic illness in late life.
    d. The rate of chronic illness exceeds acute illness until the seventh decade of life, when it then begins to decline.

13. *Which health problems occur less frequently among older persons?*

    a. Parasites and infections
    b. Breast cancer and arthritis
    c. Congestive heart failure (CHF) and transient ischemic attack (TIA)
    d. Aphasia and lung cancer

14. *Some theorists believe lipofuscin has a role in the aging process. The rationale for their thinking is:*

    a. People who ingest high levels of lipofuscin are shown to have more health problems and age at a faster rate
    b. With advanced age, older people show increasing amounts of this element in their urine samples
    c. Lipofuscin particles accumulate in certain body organs in greater amounts with advancing age
    d. Mammals and reptiles accumulate the same amount of lipofuscin in their bodies each year

15. *A community leader advocates the development of a retirement community on the outskirts of town, removed from the general population, in which the elderly could have their needs met without ever having to leave. This type of thinking is most consistent with which psychological theory of aging?*

    a. Disengagement
    b. Continuity
    c. Activity
    d. Developmental

16. *Your elderly neighbor often speaks about his accomplishments in earlier years. According to Erickson's model, you would interpret this as:*

    a. A sign of withdrawal from current stresses
    b. Depression
    c. A regressive coping mechanism
    d. A therapeutic activity

17. *Sixty-six-year-old Mr. L has just retired and asks your advice about what he should do with all his time. Your most appropriate response would be to:*

   a. Review his interests and guide him in using them to establish new roles
   b. Suggest that he develop a plan to share household chores equally with his wife
   c. Tell him to take it easy and try to develop a slower-paced life
   d. Say nothing and understand that his feelings will pass in time

18. *Which activity would not be consistent with Peck's description of developmental tasks?*

   a. Substituting new roles for lost ones
   b. Finding social and psychological satisfaction despite physical discomforts
   c. Achieving satisfaction by reflecting on one's past accomplishments
   d. Focusing on the realities of impending death

19. *Although she has been resting for 45 minutes after an active physical therapy session, 73-year-old Mrs. K continues to have an elevated pulse rate. Your most appropriate action would be to:*

   a. Do nothing and evaluate her in a few hours
   b. Massage her carotid arteries
   c. Obtain an electrocardiogram and call the physician
   d. Suggest that she perform a physical exercise

20. *You know that based on Mrs. K's situation in the aforementioned example, she should be advised to:*

   a. Avoid active physical therapy
   b. Rest between activity
   c. Follow an activity immediately with another
   d. Massage her own carotid arteries during physical activity

21. *Seventy-four-year-old Mr. T and his 30-year-old grandson attend a community health fair and have their blood pressures taken. They both are concerned when Mr. T's blood pressure is found to be 170/85, and his grandson's is 120/60. Your best advice to them should be:*

    a. Not to be alarmed as this is not abnormal
    b. Not to be alarmed, but to have their physician evaluate Mr. T's blood pressure
    c. Suggest that Mr. T get his blood pressure treated
    d. Privately tell the grandson to have Mr. T visit his physician

22. *A nursing student wants to initiate breathing exercises for a nursing home resident to aid in improving respirations, and asks your advice. You know that based on the elderly's usual respiratory changes, it would be best to:*

    a. Have an expiration to inspiration ratio of 3:1
    b. Focus more on inspirations
    c. Avoid deep respirations
    d. Avoid these exercises altogether

23. *Which is not associated with normal aging of the gastrointestinal tract?*

    a. Reduction in taste sensation
    b. Loss of teeth
    c. Decrease in gastric acid secretion
    d. Delayed emptying time of stomach

24. *Mr. J tells you he is constipated. Your initial step would be to:*

    a. Administer a bulk-forming laxative
    b. Do a rectal exam
    c. Ask him why he believes he is constipated
    d. Ignore his comment, but monitor his bowel habits

25. *Which description of bladder function would you believe to be a normal finding in late life?*

    a. Retention with anuria for as long as 24 hours
    b. Occasional incontinence

c. Lack of sensation of need to void
d. Frequency and nocturia

26. *During the home health nurse's visit, 72-year-old Mrs. M experiences an incontinent episode. Although Mrs. M has never complained of it before, upon questioning her, the nurse learns that Mrs. M has had incontinence for five to six months, but has never told any professional caring for her. You know that the most likely reason for Mrs. M's not sharing this problem is:*

a. Altered mental status
b. Lack of discomfort or distress over the problem
c. Acceptance as a normal consequence of aging
d. Desire to use this is an attention-getting measure

27. *Which could be considered an abnormality of sexual function in the elderly?*

a. Desire for masturbation
b. Difficulty of penile penetration into the vagina
c. Reduced frequency of intercourse
d. Lack of reproductive ability in the male

28. *The most significant obstacle preventing some older women from being sexually active is:*

a. Lack of a partner
b. Lack of knowledge
c. Inability to have orgasms
d. Vaginal atrophy

29. *Which is a visual change related to normal aging?*

a. Color blindness
b. Wider range of peripheral vision
c. Farsightedness
d. Blind spots in visual field

30. *Your 78-year-old nursing home resident complains that she doesn't like going outdoors on bright, sunny days because she*

can't see as well. You would recognize this to be associated with:
   a. Presbyopia
   b. Glaucoma
   c. Early detached retina
   d. Cataracts

31. *Which situation could result from a normal age-related change in vision?*
   a. Tripping while walking up the stairs
   b. Seeing halos around lights
   c. Not being able to see a dark wood door against a yellow wall
   d. Ignoring objects placed in the center of the visual field

32. *The most effective approach to communicating with individuals who have a high frequency hearing loss is to:*
   a. Have them use a hearing aid
   b. Speak in a loud, low-pitched voice
   c. Use a soft, whisper-like voice
   d. Teach them to use sign language

33. *Which statement most accurately explains why fever may appear atypically among the elderly?*
   a. Fever does not occur with infections.
   b. Normal body temperature may be lower.
   c. Temperature elevation can occur without cause.
   d. More often, hypothermia occurs with infection.

34. *A 74-year-old participant in a geriatric day care program tells you that she sponge bathes daily and takes a tub bath only twice a week. Your best action would be to:*
   a. Schedule her for daily tub baths at the center
   b. Tell her to use alcohol for cleansing her skin during her daily sponge baths
   c. Do nothing
   d. Ask her why she won't bathe more frequently

35. *Sixty-four-year-old Mrs. F tells you she is concerned about the increasing number of "age spots" that have been appearing on her arms and hands. Your best response to her is:*

    a. "These are perfectly harmless."
    b. "You should have them biopsied."
    c. "Begin taking a vitamin supplement."
    d. "Blot them with bleach several times a day."

36. *A body change that seems to support the impact of radiation on the body's aging process is:*

    a. Melanocyte clustering
    b. Senile keratoses
    c. Osteoporosis
    d. Solar elastosis

37. *A friend expresses concern to you regarding her 75-year-old mother's insomnia, stating that her mother goes to bed at 9 p.m., but can be heard walking around the house and fixing snacks in the kitchen at 4 a.m. She asks your advice on how to help her mother. Your best response would be to tell her to:*

    a. Supply a protein-rich snack immediately before her mother goes to bed
    b. Obtain a comprehensive physical and mental examination of her mother
    c. Give her mother two aspirin and warm milk at bedtime
    d. Do nothing if her mother is not bothered

38. *The diet of the older adult should consist of:*

    a. More calories of higher quality
    b. Double the vitamin and iron intake
    c. Fewer calories of higher nutritional value
    d. Higher amounts of protein, vitamins, and minerals; no fats

39. *The most important reason for nursing assessment of the older adult is:*

    a. To identify nursing problems
    b. To detect medical problems missed by the physician

    c. To fulfill regulatory requirements

    d. To determine level of care for reimbursement

40. *Which older person is at lowest risk for hypothermia?*

    a. A surgical patient in the recovery room

    b. A thin individual who never shivers

    c. A woman who shivers a lot

    d. A person who consumes a moderate amount of alcohol

41. *Which statement is true regarding myocardial infarctions in the elderly?*

    a. Chest pain may not always occur.

    b. They seldom occur in the absence of a history of cardiac disease.

    c. Few elderly survive them.

    d. Oxygen is not used in the treatment.

42. *The nursing assistant summons your help, and you find her trying to support an elderly patient who has fallen to the floor in a semiconscious state. This patient has a history of coronary artery disease, diabetes, and osteoporosis. The nursing assistant states that nothing unusual happened—the patient was straining to have a bowel movement and then suddenly collapsed. You could suspect this episode to be a result of:*

    a. Spontaneous fracture

    b. Hyperglycemic reaction

    c. The Valsalva maneuver

    d. Bowel obstruction

43. *Which would you not expect to be true of a stasis ulcer in older adults?*

    a. They are at greater risk of developing in diabetic or obese persons.

    b. The affected extremity will be cooler than the one without the ulcer.

    c. Most occur near the ankle.

    d. Three-fourths of them eventually make amputation necessary.

44. *Your 78-year-old patient in respiratory distress is prescribed nasal oxygen at 3 liters. A nursing student asks you why a lower level than that normally prescribed is being used when this patient is having trouble breathing. Your accurate response is:*

   a. Fewer cells in the older body place a lower demand for oxygen

   b. Higher levels of infusion irritate the fragile tissue along the nasal passage

   c. The elderly are started on small doses, which are gradually increased

   d. A higher infusion could depress respirations and lead to carbon dioxide build-up

45. *A true statement regarding tuberculosis in the elderly is:*

   a. It is usually a reactivation of an earlier infection

   b. Increased immunity to the disease is developed with age

   c. Tuberculin skin tests are not effective in older persons

   d. It becomes less of a problem in old age

46. *Persons with a ruddy, pink complexion who are labelled "pink puffers" can be best believed to possess which of these diseases?*

   a. Pulmonary edema

   b. Chronic bronchitis

   c. Emphysema

   d. Pneumonia

47. *In performing postural drainage for an older person, you would do all of the following except:*

   a. Administer the prescribed aerosal medication prior to the postural drainage

   b. Perform the procedure before meals

   c. Use more forceful chest pounding to loosen secretions

   d. Change positions slowly

48. *Your 66-year-old neighbor tells you he has just been diagnosed as having a hiatal hernia and asks you how he can manage this problem. You would be correct in recommending that he:*

a. Eat several, smaller meals throughout the day, rather than the three large ones he currently eats
b. Consume a large dairy product snack within a half-hour before retiring to bed
c. Use an antacid every four hours
d. Sleep in a perfectly flat position

49. *Your 82-year-old patient complains of abdominal discomfort and diarrhea. In examining her, you note that she has abdominal fullness, is lethargic, and has fecal matter on her nightgown; her appetite has been poor for several days. What would be the wisest course of action you could take?*

a. Perform a rectal examination
b. Collect a stool specimen for culture
c. Obtain an order for an antidiarrheal drug
d. Keep her NPO for the next 24 hours until the physician can examine her tomorrow

50. *Dr. J tells you not to bother testing the urine of his elderly diabetic patient because he prefers having her blood glucose evaluated. Why would he be selecting blood tests over urine samples?*

a. Older persons can be hyperglycemic without spilling glucose into their urines.
b. Clinitest and other urine testing methods are not sensitive to the elderly's urine.
c. Glucose in the blood is more stable than glucose in the urine.
d. There is no rationale for his preference.

51. *Which statement is not true regarding glucose tolerance testing in older adults?*

a. Age-related gradients are used in interpreting the test.
b. Large doses of salicylates can reduce blood glucose and alter results.
c. Older adults can have a normal fasting blood glucose but be hyperglycemic after carbohydrate intake.
d. Carbohydrates are eliminated from the diet several days before testing.

52. *Your 69-year-old patient asks to be taken to the bathroom every 15 minutes. Your best reaction would be:*
   a. Tell her she needn't toilet so frequently, as her bladder can actually hold more urine
   b. Ask her why she needs to toilet so frequently and if she voids each time she toilets
   c. Toilet her, recognizing this as a normal consequence of aging
   d. Toilet her every two hours and have her wear an adult diaper

53. *The laboratory indicates that a slight elevation in bacteria was found in Mrs. D's urine. You are surprised because she has shown no signs indicating a urinary tract infection. Mrs. D's physician is informed and states that he chooses not to treat her at this time, but will push fluids and monitor her. The reason for the physician's nontreatment can best be explained by:*
   a. Prescribing antibiotics would encourage a new strain of bacteria to emerge
   b. Physicians generally lack interest in older patients
   c. Antibiotics are not effective in treating urinary tract infections in the elderly
   d. A majority of older people have some degree of urinary tract infection

54. *Which is an accurate statement regarding prostatic hypertrophy in old age?*
   a. Black males have twice the rate of white males.
   b. Most prostatic surgeries do not cause impotency.
   c. Incontinence is a primary sign.
   d. Most cases develop into malignancies.

55. *"Hot flashes" in aging women:*
   a. Result from lowered estrogen levels
   b. Are associated with cardiovascular changes having nothing to do with the reproductive system

    c. Are of greater prevalence among women who have had
       multiple pregnancies
    d. Have no physiological basis

56. *A nurse friend who is employed in a gynecologist's practice
tells you that she has recently seen several older women in the
office being treated for vaginitis and asks you if there is any
special reason for this. Your most accurate response would be:*

    a. The more alkaline secretions of the older female's vagina
       place her at higher risk of infection
    b. In older women, this is a common precancerous sign
    c. This is usually associated with estrogen replacement therapy
    d. This is an extremely rare occurrence

57. *Mrs. S has a history of glaucoma. Which sign would indicate
that Mrs. S is experiencing an increase in her intraocular pressure?*

    a. Cloudy lens
    b. Loss of color vision
    c. Absence of tearing
    d. Dull headaches

58. *Which of the following would most likely precipitate a transient ischemic attack in a person with a history of this problem?*

    a. Quickly rising from a lying to a standing position
    b. Administration of aspirin on a regular basis
    c. Reduction in activity level
    d. Rapid change in weather conditions

59. *In examining a 68-year-old woman, you detect bony nodules
on the joints of several of her fingers. You could suspect this to be
associated with:*

    a. Rheumatoid arthritis
    b. Osteoporosis
    c. Osteoarthritis
    d. Paget's disease

60. *Which would not be a contributing factor in the development of gout?*

   a. Underexcretion of uric acid
   b. Overproduction of uric acid
   c. Insulin therapy
   d. Thiazide diuretic therapy

61. *Next to the hip, a common site of fractures in the elderly is the:*

   a. Wrist
   b. Skull
   c. Rib cage
   d. Ankle

62. *A patient on your unit returns from physical therapy with a cane to assist in his ambulation. You would know that the correct use of this cane consists of positioning it on:*

   a. The affected side and advancing it with the affected leg
   b. The affected side and advancing it with the unaffected leg
   c. The unaffected side and advancing it with the affected leg
   d. The unaffected side and advancing it with the unaffected leg

63. *You are assisting a wheelchair-bound person who has right-sided weakness in returning to bed. Your appropriate positioning of the wheelchair is to place it so that the:*

   a. The patient's right side is next to the bed
   b. The patient's left side is next to the bed
   c. The chair is facing the bed, approximately two feet away
   d. The chair is parallel to the foot of the bed

64. *During the mental status examination portion of the assessment, you request the client to do all of the items described in a-d below. Which one is the best test of the client's judgment?*

   a. Pick up the paper, fold it in half, and hand it to me
   b. Place the page in the holes as quickly as you can
   c. Explain what is meant by "A bird in the hand is worth two in the bush"
   d. Count backwards from 100 by 7's

65. *Seventy-three-year-old Mrs. R comes to the clinic accompanied by her daughter. The daughter states that Mrs. R has seemed confused lately. Your best response is to:*

    a. Send Mrs. R for a complete physical examination
    b. Interview Mrs. R and her daughter to learn more about her possible confusion
    c. Recognize this as the daughter's anxiety and reassure her that there is probably nothing wrong
    d. Arrange for a home visit by the mental health nurse

66. *With which condition can depression sometimes be easily mistaken?*

    a. Anxiety
    b. Alcoholism
    c. Delirium
    d. Dementia

67. *Seventy-year-old Mr. O is the husband of one of your nursing home residents. His wife has been institutionalized for eight years and is in stable condition. Mr. O has maintained the family home during that time, although he has barely met his expenses. Last month he sold his car because of a significant rise in his insurance. Mr. O's daughter drives him to the facility for visits now, and during one of the visits she tells you that her father hasn't been himself lately; he is moping around, not eating his favorite foods that she prepares for him, losing interest in his appearance, and is generally, acting depressed. If Mr. O is depressed, it would most likely be associated with:*

    a. His wife's condition
    b. Limited finances
    c. Household burdens
    d. Ceasing to drive

68. *Which group has the highest rate of suicide?*

    a. White males over age 75
    b. Late stage Alzheimer's victims
    c. Black males ages 65-75
    d. White widows over age 70

69. *Mr. C is visiting the mental health clinic for assessment of his dementia. Halfway through the routine interview, he becomes hostile and refuses to answer any more questions. Your best action is to:*

   a. Discontinue the interview
   b. Ignore his reaction and proceed
   c. Ask him if he is feeling insulted or embarrassed by the questions being asked
   d. Explain to him that this information will help in planning individualized care for him

70. *One of the nursing home residents with multi-infarct dementia has asked for the time several times in the past hour. On her next request for the time, your best response would be to:*

   a. Tell her the time
   b. Tell her you have told her the time and to try to remember what you told her
   c. Ask her why she continues asking the same question
   d. Tell her she is annoying others by asking for the time

71. *The most important environmental factor in aiding the function of Alzheimer's victims is:*

   a. Variety
   b. Unrestricted wandering
   c. High stimulation
   d. Consistency

72. *You visit Mrs. B three weeks after her husband's death. Her sister, widowed five years ago, is with her and you find them both crying. The sister tells you that she can sympathize with Mrs. B because she too was married almost 50 years and still thinks about her husband all the time; she claims she is unable to sleep through the night without crying over his death. Mrs. B shakes her head in agreement and says, "Yes, that is how it is with me." Your best response to Mrs. B would be:*

   a. It is normal to feel this way so soon after your husband's death; in time, these feelings will lessen.
   b. You shouldn't keep grieving your loss, but get on with your own life.

    c. You'd be better off giving yourself time alone and not listening to other widows.
    d. Although the pain you are feeling will be a constant part of your life, you must try to find happiness.

73. *In the aforementioned situation, you recognize Mrs. B's sister's grief to be:*

    a. Unresolved and abnormal
    b. A normal reaction to a long, happy marriage that has ended
    c. An attention-getting mechanism
    d. A compensation for the poor relationship she had with her husband while he was alive

74. *Widowed Mr. W spends most of his day in activities related to his pet dog. He takes the dog for long walks, cooks a full dinner that the dog gets a portion of, and is constantly writing his children anecdotes about the dog's latest pranks. Your best reaction to the situation would be to:*

    a. Counsel Mr. W to focus the same attention on a human being rather than a dog
    b. Obtain a mental status evaluation
    c. Contact his children to discuss ways to expand his social world
    d. Do nothing

75. *A general rule of thumb regarding geriatric pharmacology is:*

    a. Except for cardiac drugs, all medications should be prescribed in greater amounts
    b. Drugs are less effective in late life
    c. Most drugs do more harm than good
    d. Lower doses of most medications should be used

76. *One problem with using acetaminophen in the management of arthritis is:*

    a. It lacks an anti-inflammatory effect
    b. A tolerance can develop
    c. It is not an effective analgesic in the elderly
    d. It can exacerbate joint pain as a potential side effect

77. *Mr. R tells you he has been taking his digoxin with an antacid to prevent heartburn. You recognize that:*

a. This is a sound practice
b. The effects of digoxin can be increased
c. The effects of digoxin can be decreased
d. There will be no positive or negative effects from the antacid

78. *Mrs. U uses miotic eye drops for her glaucoma. She is scheduled for orthopedic surgery. You know that the eye drops should:*

a. Not be administered two days prior to surgery but can be used immediately postoperatively
b. Not be used two days before or two days after surgery
c. Be administered without interruption
d. Be discontinued until her discharge from the hospital

79. *Mr. H has been using mineral oil as a laxative daily over the past several months. Which of the following problems that he displays would be least likely to be associated with the use of mineral oil?*

a. Respiratory infections
b. Vitamin A and D deficiencies
c. Diarrhea
d. Fat particles in stool

80. *Mr. T is using nitroglycerin ointment. In discussing his application of the ointment, he tells you that he uses the same site at all times (a hairless part of his arm), thoroughly removes all old ointment before the new application is made, and leaves the ointment on, untouched until the next application. The one change to Mr. T's procedure that you would recommend would be to:*

a. Apply the ointment to the chest or abdomen rather than to the arm
b. Not wash off the former application
c. Use different application sites each day
d. Thoroughly remove the ointment four hours after application

81. *Probenecid is effective in the treatment of gout by:*

   a. Inhibiting the kidney tubules' reabsorption of uric acid
   b. Inhibiting inflammation
   c. Depressing CNS function
   d. Relaxing muscle tissue

82. *Mr. L is demonstrating involuntary rhythmic movements of his tongue, face, and limbs. Of the following medications he is receiving, which would be associated with this problem?*

   a. Digoxin
   b. Chloral hydrate
   c. Haloperidol
   d. Levodopa

83. *Which would you know to be a true statement regarding older nursing home residents?*

   a. There are the same number of older persons in psychiatric hospitals as in nursing homes.
   b. Most nursing home residents are widowed females.
   c. Only a small minority of nursing home residents have a mental illness.
   d. Most are private-pay patients.

84. *The most significant factor believed to be responsible for the growth of nursing home beds is:*

   a. Increased number of elderly persons
   b. Decreased responsibility of families for care of the older relatives
   c. Passage of Medicare and Medical Assistance legislation in the 1960s
   d. Greater societal acceptance of this form of care

85. *In looking at future service needs of the older population, which would not be likely?*

   a. The elderly will have fewer health problems and service needs.
   b. More nursing home beds will be needed.

c. Families will be providing more direct care for longer periods of time.
d. The elderly will be paying for more services out of their own pockets.

86. *Which among the following is the most important factor in determining an older person's risk of institutionalization?*
    a. Available family support
    b. Ability to pay
    c. Number of medical problems
    d. Desire of the individual

87. *A new staff member feels it would be uplifting and invigorating to the residents of the nursing home for the residents to change their rooms and roommates. Your best response to this suggestion is:*
    a. "There is a risk of more negative than positive outcomes from this type of change."
    b. "All of the residents will have some type of physical reaction from this move."
    c. "This type of change is known to improve the functional capacity of nursing home residents."
    d. "This type of change has been shown to have benefit for residents and staff."

88. *You receive a call from the son of one of your nursing home residents who tells you that his father is writing letters to family members telling them that the son is "an inconsiderate, greedy liar who is just interested in his inheritance." The son says he is embarrassed by his father's behavior and asks that you take his father's letters from the outgoing mail bin and give them to the son before they can be mailed. Your appropriate action should be:*
    a. Follow the son's request
    b. Read all the letters before they are mailed and include an explanatory note if a letter is inflammatory
    c. Continue to allow the letters to be mailed
    d. Refuse to supply writing paper to the resident and ask him to speak with his son about the matter

89. *Which is not an accurate statement regarding elder abuse?*

    a. It can consist of physical, psychological, financial, or sexual acts.
    b. There are laws protecting the elderly from abuse.
    c. Most abuse is committed by persons close to the older adult.
    d. Older individuals readily report their abuse once they are aware of the reporting procedure.

90. *You are the evening supervisor in a small nursing home. You notice that one of your patients is coughing and has a low-grade fever. You call the physician and say that you believe the patient is developing pneumonia. The physician gives a telephone order for an antibiotic and says he will visit the patient first thing tomorrow. During the night, the patient's condition worsens and he dies en route to the hospital from what is later determined to be a myocardial infarction. The family brings a lawsuit against you and the physician. In terms of liability:*

    a. You and the physician can be held responsible for malpractice
    b. Only the physician is responsible
    c. Only you are responsible
    d. Only the facility can be sued

91. *The physician is concerned that 72-year-old Mrs. J will be upset if the need for her surgery is fully explained to her and consults with Mr. J to obtain consent for surgery. Mr. J tells the physician to obtain consent from their son who "is better able to understand these things." In reference to this consent, you know that:*

    a. Mrs. J must grant consent
    b. Only the next of kin can grant consent, which in this case would be Mr. J
    c. Any blood relative can grant consent, if the patient will be disturbed by the explanation of the procedure
    d. The physician should obtain consent from Mrs. J, but omit explaining the procedure and its risks

92. *Medicare is a:*

    a. Program of no-cost health insurance for persons age 65 and over, and for the poor of all ages
    b. Contributory health insurance program for persons age 65 and over
    c. Health insurance program for the poor of all ages
    d. Federal health insurance program for persons unable to qualify for private health insurance

93. *Medicare reimburses for:*

    a. Only hospital bills
    b. Hospital and physician bills
    c. Hospital and physician bills and unlimited nursing home care
    d. Medical, surgical, dental, and nursing care in any Medicare participating agency

94. *Which is a valid statement regarding the regulation of health care practice?*

    a. Local city and county governments do not have the authority to develop regulations.
    b. Federal regulations are optional if state regulations exist.
    c. Agencies who accept only private-pay patients are exempt from regulations.
    d. State regulations can be more stringent than federal regulations.

95. *Which of the following would you not recognize as part of the ANA Standards for Gerontological Nursing?*

    a. Data are systematically and continuously collected about the health status of the older adult.
    b. A plan of nursing care is developed according to the prescribed medical plan.
    c. The plan of nursing care includes priorities and prescribed nursing approaches.
    d. The older adult and significant others participate in determining progress attained in achieving goals.

96. *The basic foundations upon which a strong quality assurance program is built are:*

    a. Audits
    b. Standards
    c. Policies and procedures
    d. QA plans

97. *A director of nursing wants to determine if all medications given over the past month have been signed by a licensed nurse at the appropriate times. This type of audit is:*

    a. Structure
    b. Outcome
    c. Concurrent
    d. Process

98. *The staff want to initiate a 15 minute/day exercise program with a select group of elderly to see if there will be any decrease in their arthritis symptoms. To determine if the desired results are being achieved, you would want to conduct which type of audit?*

    a. Structure
    b. Outcome
    c. Retrospective
    d. Process

99. *One major problem of past gerontological research has been:*

    a. Insufficient studies of institutionalized populations
    b. High proportion of replicated studies
    c. Too much reliance on conceptual models
    d. Poor methodology

100. *Which is an accurate statement about the ANA's Gerontological Nursing Division?*

    a. It was one of the earliest specialty divisions.
    b. It was officially formed in 1966.
    c. It was once part of the American Geriatrics Society.
    d. It is considered a subspecialty of the medical-surgical nursing division.

PART II:

Test Answers and Discussion

Test Answers and Discussion

The preceding 100 questions offer a sampling of the subjects included in the ANA Certification Examination. Knowledge of these subjects is essential to gerontological nursing practice. This section will discuss the responses by identifying the correct answer and explaining why the other responses were incorrect. After reviewing the responses and evaluating your performance on the test, it can be beneficial to identify any patterns associated with incorrect responses, e.g., not having read the entire question before responding, overlooking key words such as *not* or *all but,* or selecting the first reasonable sounding answer without reading through all the responses for the best selection. When incorrect responses are associated with knowledge deficits, it is advisable to explore some of the literature listed under the specific heading in the bibliography section.

Facts About The Older Population

Demographics

1. *Which statement best describes the older population in the United States?*
    a. It is predominantly male.
    b. It is comprised of greater numbers of "old-old."
    c. It is becoming a smaller percentage of the total population.
    d. It is enjoying a longer lifespan than previous generations.

The elderly population is becoming an older one because more people than ever are surviving to their eighth decade and beyond. In 1930, when there were slightly more than six million persons over the age of 65, the life expectancy was 59.7 years; by 1965 life expectancy increased to 70.2 years, and the number of elderly swelled to over 20 million. Today, the life expectancy is 74.7 years, and there are more than 27 million older adults, representing almost 12 percent of the total population of our country. It is predicted that at the turn of the century, 20 percent of the United States population will be over age 65 (U.S. Bureau of the Census 1986a).

Improved living conditions and health care have not only helped more people survive to old age, but have facilitated them to live longer once they become senior citizens. In 1960, 10.4 million individuals were over the age of 70; in 1983 that segment of the population grew to 18.5 million. The number of persons age 85 and older nearly tripled within that time, going from 0.9 million to 2.5 million. That trend will continue, and we will see more "old-old" persons in our society.

The older population is not predominantly male. Women enjoy a life expectancy of more than eight years greater than their male counterparts. In fact, over the years, the ratio of male to female in late life has decreased. With each advancing decade of life, the ratio of male to female further declines.

With all this talk of people living longer, you may wonder why *d* was not the correct answer. True, life expectancy (the average number of years one can expect to live) has increased, but lifespan (the total number of years the human organism is capable of living) has not changed.

2. *You relocate to a new state and are interested in working with older adults in the community. In surveying available services, you discover that most geriatric programs are located in urban areas. The most likely reason for this is:*

   a. City governments have placed higher priority on the elderly than county governments
   b. Rural and suburban elderly are less responsive to formal services than urban elderly
   c. Families in rural and suburban areas provide more services to older relatives than those in urban areas
   d. The largest number of elderly are found in urban areas

The largest number of older adults reside in cities, with the next greatest amount in rural areas. Only a small proportion of suburban residents are over the age of 65, although that is changing as the young couples who moved to suburbia in the 1950s and 1960s are now entering their senior years. The top ranking states for possessing the highest *percentage* of elderly residents are Florida, Rhode Island, Iowa, and Pennsylvania, although the states with the greatest *numbers* of seniors are California, New York, Pennsylvania, and Texas. States with a low percentage of their total population being over age 65 include Alaska, Utah, Wyoming, and Hawaii. Service provision has been more a reflection of where the elderly are than anything else. There is no evidence to support that cities place a greater priority on geriatric services than counties, or that the elderly in one area are more responsive to services than older persons in other areas. Availability, accessibility, and affordability play more significant roles in service utilization. Regardless of geographic area, families are increasingly more involved with their elder members.

3. Which situation is most typical of the living arrangements of most older adults?

    a. An older man living in a rooming house alone
    b. Two sisters sharing an apartment
    c. A married couple living in the community
    d. A widow living in her children's home

Although elderly persons can be found in any of the aforementioned living arrangements, the most typical of the choices offered would be *c*. Less than one in seven older men live alone, and approximately 18 percent of all older women are living with any relative other than a spouse (less than 6 percent for older males). Approximately 10 percent of older women and 5 percent of older men live with children and grandchildren. Thus, a married couple living in the community is the correct answer. Although more than half of the elderly are living with a spouse, the differences for the sexes must be recognized: more than half of all older women are widowed, while more than three-fourths of all older men have a living spouse. The practice of women marrying men older than themselves and the longer life expectancy of women contribute to the high ratio of widows to widowers. The widowed or single older woman living alone is at greatest risk of institutionalization.

4. A group of neighbors ranging in ages from 64 to 76 meet for lunch weekly. All of the women are widowed. Which statement best describes their widowhood?

    a. They are atypical of most older women.
    b. They represent the reality for most older women.

c. Few women in their age group are widowed.

d. They are outnumbered by widowers at that age.

The answer to question three should have explained this.

5. *You are leading a discussion group for middle-aged persons who wish to learn more about their elderly parents. As the participants share their own family experiences, which statement would you recognize as describing an unusual situation?*

a. "My parents and I live within a half-hour of each other, and we all prefer that arrangement."

b. "My mother and father had a rocky marriage for years, but now they seem to have calmed down and get along better."

c. "My parents and I are in touch at least once a week."

d. "My mother and her sister used to be close, but they now have drifted apart."

Contrary to the prevailing myth that families neglect or avoid contact with their elder members, most older adults do have regular contact, at least once during the week. Children do assist older parents with shopping, finances, home maintenance, and other functions, and in turn, often receive assistance from their parents. Although caring and involvement exist, most elderly and their children prefer having separate residences, ideally within a half-hour distance from one another.

As for marriage in late life, even the stormiest marital relationship stabilizes. Most couples overlook the shortcomings and disappointments as they share new challenges that strengthen their interdependency. Although the numbers have been increasing, couples who divorce in late life remain in the minority.

If *a, b,* and *c* are not unusual situations, the most uncommon situation must be *d*. Siblings may drift apart through their adult years as they become absorbed in their separate families, interests, and careers; however, they typically grow closer in old age and form a bond that comes second only to that between parent and child.

Cultural Aspects

6. *As compared with white elderly, older blacks*

a. Do not live as long, but have strong family ties.
b. Are poorer, although healthier.
c. Have a male life expectancy that exceeds that of females.
d. Have a higher rate of institutionalization.

A history of poorer standards of living, less access to health care, and special hardships unique to blacks, have contributed to black Americans' having poorer health and a lower life expectancy (National Center for Health Statistics 1986, 69):

Life Expectancy in Years

	White	Black
Female	77.2	71.2
Male	69.4	62.9

As the table shown above illustrates, the lowest life expectancy in the United States is among black males.

Income also is lower among older blacks who have more than $5,000 less annual income per capita than older whites and more than three times the number of persons living with incomes below the poverty level.

Black families provide strong support and caregiving functions to their elders, who are viewed with high esteem. This factor contributes to the lower rate of institutionalization among blacks. (Past discriminatory practices and economic limitations were factors, as well.)

7. *You are a new public health nurse on an American Indian reservation. In establishing priorities for the health screening of this group, the high-risk problem that you would be most interested in addressing is:*

a. Violence
b. Tuberculosis
c. Alcoholism
d. Pancreatic cancer

There are nearly one million Indians in the U.S. who constitute the 493 recognized tribes in this country. Indians suffered as new settlers invaded their land, and experienced prejudicial treatment throughout the years. Despite efforts by the federal government to assist the

American Indians, high unemployment and social pressures created stresses leading to alcohol abuse. Alcoholism is a serious problem among the Indian population and is of greater risk to this group than any of the other problems listed among the responses.

8. *Which is true regarding older Orientals in the U.S.?*

    a. They are held in high esteem by their families.
    b. Most have settled in New York.
    c. They have experienced very little prejudice.
    d. There is a higher female:male ratio among older Chinese than among the non-Oriental elderly.

Large scale immigration of Chinese and Japanese people was most evident in the latter part of the 17th century when poor conditions in their home countries led them to America to earn a better living. These immigrants were willing to work for substandard wages, making them disliked among American workers. Prejudicial treatment resulted, demonstrated through restrictions on immigration quotas, property ownership, and Oriental-American marriages. Despite the prejudices they faced, Orientals have a lower rate of unemployment and a higher percentage of professionals than the general population. California seems to be the state where most Orientals settled and remained.

Many Chinese men immigrated to this country with the hopes of earning enough money to return to their homes or send for their families to join them in America. The prejudice and low wages they confronted prevented them from actualizing their goals, and most of these Chinese men remained single, giving them the unique display of more older men than women. Just the opposite is true for the Japanese men who had young brides sent to them from their country, thus creating a higher proportion of Japanese widows than is seen in the non-Oriental population.

The Orientals possess strong family bonds, and elder relatives are viewed with reverence. The old are sought for advice and influence family decisions, although this is slowly changing. It is expected that the family will care for its older members.

9. *As a new public health nurse, you find that there are many Hispanics in your community, and you wish to address their unique*

interests and needs. Which of the following actions would be most appropriate for this group?

    a. Helping them establish a nursing home in their community.
    b. Developing caregiver education and support.
    c. Suspending home visits from sundown Friday to sunrise Saturday.
    d. Utilizing lay healers.

Individuals from Spain and the Latin American countries and their descendants are described by the term Hispanic. Most Hispanics are highly religious people who view health status as an outcome of God's actions. Therefore, prayer and religious articles play a large part in staying well and managing illness. These individuals have great respect for their elderly and see old age as the time to harvest the rewards of life. Nursing home care is not welcomed and is used as the last resort; nursing home utilization for Hispanics is lower than the average for the general population. Families feel a responsibility to care for their elders; indeed, children are viewed as a strong resource for one's later years. Thus, helping family caregivers provide that care through education and support would be your most helpful action as a nurse working with this group.

Financial Aspects

10. *What is the primary source of income for most older individuals?*

    a. Employment earnings
    b. Private pensions
    c. Social Security
    d. Investment income

When it was enacted in 1935, Social Security was intended to supplement other sources of income in old age. For most elderly, however, Social Security is the primary source of income. Labor statistics reveal that less than 3 percent of the labor force is comprised of persons over age 65. Only a minority, although a growing number, of elderly receive income from private pensions or investments.

11. *Regarding the financial status of the elderly, which is a true statement?*

    a. Older women possess more wealth and income than their male counterparts.
    b. The percentage of elderly in the poverty level has been steadily declining.
    c. There is no significant difference between the income of black and white elderly.
    d. A majority of retirees have incomes from private pension plans.

There are significant income differences between the sexes and races in old age. As discussed in question six, black elderly have the lowest incomes and highest rate of poverty among the older population. Most of today's older women lack an employment history that could have provided pension income and often find their income significantly reduced upon the death of their spouses; only a minority possess independent wealth. Also, as mentioned in the preceding question, only a minority of retirees enjoy private pensions, and most pension income is less than one-half that of employed years. Although economic conditions are not ideal, they have been steadily improving for the elderly. In 1960, over 35 percent of the elderly had incomes below the poverty level; that number has now shrunk to approximately 14 percent (U.S. Bureau of the Census 1986 b). It is felt that the number of older adults living in poverty would appear to be even less if housing, food, health, and other types of subsidies were factored in. It is believed that there will be a continued trend of fewer elderly living with poverty level incomes.

Rates of Illness

12. *Which statement would you know to be a fact regarding the rate of illness in old age?*

    a. Chronic illness occurs at four times the rate as in younger years, while acute illness occurs at one-half the rate.
    b. Acute and chronic illness occur at the same rate.

 c. The rate of acute illness begins to exceed the rate of chronic illness in late life.

 d. The rate of chronic illness exceeds acute illness until the seventh decade of life, when it then begins to decline.

Most people are aware that health problems increase with age, but many fail to recognize that this is not true for all types of illnesses. Chronic illness occurs at a rate four times higher than in persons under age 65; 80 percent of all older adults have at least one chronic illness, with the typical pattern being several chronic problems that must be managed simultaneously. The 10 major chronic illnesses affecting the elderly and their rates for younger adults are shown below:

10 Major Chronic Illnesses and Rates for Adults

per 1000 persons

	7- 44 years	45 - 64 years	65+years
Arthritis	47.7	246.5	464.7
Hypertension	54.2	243.7	378.6
Hearing impairments	43.8	142.9	283.8
Heart conditions	37.9	122.7	277.0
Chronic sinusitis	158.4	177.5	183.6
Visual impairments	27.4	55.2	136.6
Orthopedic problems	90.5	117.5	128.2
Diabetes	8.6	56.9	83.4
Varicose veins	19.0	50.1	83.2
Hemorrhoids	43.7	66.6	65.9

(Source: U.S. National Center for Health Statistics)

The picture is different where acute illnesses are concerned. The rate for acute problems is one-half that for younger adults. Infections and injuries occur less frequently among the old. Respiratory illnesses are the most common type of acute problem; however, they are reported at a lower rate among the elderly. To persons working with the sick aged, this fact may come as a surprise because the severe effects of acute conditions in this population are often encountered. Although they occur less frequently, acute problems result in higher rates of complications and mortality when they are present; thus, they remain a serious threat to the elderly.

13.*Which health problems occur less frequently among older persons?*

    a. Parasites and infections
    b. Breast cancer and arthritis
    c. Congestive heart failure (CHF) and transient ischemic attack (TIA)
    d. Aphasia and lung cancer

The previous question explains why the only response with acute problems would be correct. The other three responses not only contain chronic problems, but include those that are the major causes of death for older persons: heart disease, cancer, and stroke.

Theories of Aging

Biological Aging

14. *Some theorists believe lipofuscin has a role in the aging process. The rationale for their thinking is:*

    a. People who ingest high levels of lipofuscin are shown to have more health problems and age at a faster rate
    b. With advanced age, older people show increasing amounts of this element in their urine samples
    c. Lipofuscin particles accumulate in certain body organs in greater amounts with advancing age
    d. Mammals and reptiles accumulate the same amount of lipofuscin in their bodies each year

Throughout history, there have been innumerable attempts to explain why humans grow old. Although no exact cause for aging is known, there are several theories that hypothesize the role of various factors in the aging process. Those theories that discuss the changes to the body's structure and function are called biological theories; those that address the aging individual's behaviors, thinking, and feelings are called psychological theories; and those that review the relationship of society to the older adult are labelled sociological theories.

A variety of biological theories exist, including those that relate aging to genetic factors, mutations of DNA, cross-linking of collagen, diet, radiation, autoimmune reactions, and stress. One theory considers the role of lipofuscin. Lipofuscin is a lipoprotein by-product of metabolism with no known function in the body; however, this material increasingly accumulates in body organs as one ages. It also appears in other species at a rate proportionate to their lifespan (i.e., if a species has one-third the lifespan as humans, it will accumulate lipofuscin at three times the rate of humans) (Few and Getty 1967). Whether it plays a role in causing aging to occur or is an outcome of this process is unclear, but the ability to quantify the relationship of aging to lipofuscin accumulation makes this a popular theory among scientists. Again, this is just a theory; to date there is no single factor known to cause or prevent the aging process.

Psychological Aging

15. *A community leader advocates the development of a retirement community on the outskirts of town, removed from the general population, in which the elderly could have their needs met without ever having to leave. This type of thinking is most consistent with which psychological theory of aging?*

   a. Disengagement
   b. Continuity
   c. Activity
   d. Developmental

One of the earliest psychological theories of aging was the Disengagement Theory, developed in the sixties by Elaine Cumming and William Henry (Cumming and Henry 1961). Basically, this theory states that it is mutually beneficial for the elderly and society to withdraw from each other. By doing so, the elderly can slow their pace and take time to reflect on their lives and center on themselves; society can transfer power and roles from the old to the young and not suffer any disruption of function. The position taken by the community leader in the above example is consistent with this theory.

The Disengagement Theory has lost popularity as people began to see that this withdrawal was not as beneficial as first believed. There are many senior citizens who thrive on staying actively involved in the mainstream of life and who contribute greatly to society (just consider the many entertainers, politicians, artists, and writers who have made significant contributions beyond their sixth decade of life). To promote mandatory retirement, segregated housing for seniors, and other measures to separate the elderly from the rest of society would be a disservice.

The Activity Theory, developed by Robert Havighurst, proposed just the opposite of disengagement. Rather than withdraw, older people should be expected to remain active in the mainstream of life, finding new roles and activities to substitute for lost ones (Havighurst 1963). Certainly, activity is more advantageous than inactivity, but to expect or force all old people to stay active may not be realistic: some elderly lack the health or resources to maintain a middle-aged life-style, while others are glad to be removed from the hustle and bustle of an active society. Gradually, this theory has lost its popularity also.

The Developmental, or Continuity Theory has now taken hold (Neugarten 1964). Bernice Neugarten, the developer of this theory, has studied the aging patterns of many individuals and found great variation. Some people welcome the chance to withdraw from the mainstream of life, while others stay actively involved as long as possible. These differences do not originate with the onset of old age; rather, they are a continuation of what their behaviors have always been: the young person who enjoyed coming home from work, shutting out the world, and curling up with a good book most likely will not become the gregarious leader of the senior center in old age; the young activist who joined every cause probably won't be sitting in a rocking chair watching the world pass her by when she becomes old.

16. *Your elderly neighbor often speaks about his accomplishments in earlier years. According to Erickson's model, you would interpret this as:*

    a. A sign of withdrawal from current stresses
    b. Depression
    c. A regressive coping mechanism
    d. A therapeutic activity

It is believed that there are certain challenges and developmental tasks, that face individuals at different stages of life. Satisfactorily fulfilling these tasks can make the difference between persons feeling good about their lives or unhappy and maladjusted. Erik Erikson described the developmental tasks during eight stages of life as (Erikson 1963):

Infancy: trust vs. mistrust
Toddler: autonomy vs. shame
Early childhood: initiative vs. guilt
Middle childhood: industry vs. inferiority
Adolescence: identity vs. identity diffusion
Adulthood: intimacy vs. isolation
Middle age: generativity vs. self-absorption
Old age: integrity vs. despair

When one reaches old age with the satisfactory achievement of each stage, there is a sense of satisfaction with one's life; despair and bitterness with one's existence grows from inadequate fulfillment of developmental tasks. Priscilla Ebersole, Irene Burnside, and Robert Butler with Myrna Lewis have described the use of "life review" or "reminiscence therapy" in their writings, and emphasize the therapeutic importance for an older person to strengthen ego integrity by discussing past accomplishments (Burnside 1984, Butler and Lewis 1982, Ebersole 1976). Gerontological nurses can foster this activity by being active and interested listeners, and helping older adults to recognize the challenges they have successfully met.

17. *Sixty-six-year-old Mr. L has just retired and asks your advice about what he should do with all his time. Your most appropriate response would be to:*

a. Review his interests and guide him in using them to establish new roles.
  b. Suggest that he develop a plan to share household chores equally with his wife.
  c. Tell him to take it easy and try to develop a slower-paced life.
  d. Say nothing and understand that his feelings will pass in time.

Significant changes and losses of roles frequently occur with advanced age. These can create a sense of profound loss, anxiety, and meaninglessness to life; physical and mental health problems can result. Your best approach as a nurse would be to assess the interests and capabilities of the individual and help him to gain new roles to replace lost ones. You wouldn't want to suggest that he assume some of his wife's chores without including her in the discussion because you could be robbing her of activities that help her in maintaining a significant role. Taking it easy and slowing down may not only be inappropriate for this man, but would also violate an important goal of gerontological care; namely, being able to maintain optimum activity. Doing nothing won't help Mr. L and could waste valuable time that could be applied to moving in a positive direction. Following the thinking of Erikson and Peck (see answer to next question), you should be aware that aiding Mr. L in establishing new roles will promote a sense of integrity within him.

18. *Which activity would not be consistent with Peck's description of developmental tasks?*

   a. Substituting new roles for lost ones.
   b. Finding social and psychological satisfaction despite physical discomforts.
   c. Achieving satisfaction by reflecting on one's past accomplishments.
   d. Focusing on the realities of impending death.

Robert Peck took Erikson's discussion of developmental tasks a stage further by outlining specific challenges that will determine whether or not a person achieves ego integrity or despair (Peck 1956, 88-92). These tasks are:

> *Ego differentiation vs. role preoccupation:* Substituting new roles for lost one
>
> *Body transcendence:* Finding psychological and social satisfactions despite physical discomforts
>
> *Ego transcendence vs. ego preoccupation:* Deriving satisfaction by reflecting on one's past, rather than becoming absorbed with the reality of one's mortality

Of the activities listed among the responses, *d* would thus be the one inconsistent with Peck's views on necessary tasks to achieve psychological satisfaction in old age.

Physical Aging and Nursing Response

Cardiovascular Changes

19. *Although she has been resting for 45 minutes after an active physical therapy session, 73-year-old Mrs. K continues to have an elevated pulse rate. Your most appropriate action would be:*
   a. Do nothing and evaluate her in a few hours
   b. Massage her carotid arteries
   c. Obtain an electrocardiogram and call the physician
   d. Suggest that she perform a physical exercise

The cardiovascular system experiences significant changes with age. Many of these changes are outcomes of one's health practices over a lifetime: persons who eat a well-balanced diet, exercise regularly, and limit the amount of stress to their bodies will not suffer the losses of those who abuse their bodies. Some of the general changes seen in many persons by the time they reach age 70 are:

- thickening and rigidity of heart valves
- less elasticity of vessels
- narrower lumen of vessels due to accumulated deposits, leading to rise in blood pressure
- reduced cardiac output

Despite these changes, most older persons fulfill their activities of daily living with no cardiac distress or discomfort. It is usually not until an extra demand is placed on the heart that these changes become evident. When faced with a stress—such as exercise or the anticipation of being examined—the older person may experience tachycardia that lasts significantly longer than it would for younger adults. Whereas a younger person's heart rate would normally return to its baseline rate within a half-hour after a stress, it may take several hours for older hearts to recover. This consideration is important in assessing the pulse of older adults: it is crucial to review the stresses experienced during previous hours whenever tachycardia is discovered.

20. *You know that based on Mrs. K's situation in the aforementioned example, she should be advised to:*

    a. Avoid active physical therapy
    b. Rest between activities
    c. Follow an activity immediately with another
    d. Massage her own carotid arteries during physical activity

Since the heart requires more time to recover from stress in old age, resting between activities is important. It isn't necessary to discontinue physical therapy in Mrs. K's situation, but to assure that it is not scheduled immediately following or preceding other activities. Massaging carotid arteries it not an appropriate intervention for Mrs. K and could lead to other problems.

21. *Seventy-four-year-old Mr. T and his 30-year-old grandson attend a community health fair and have their blood pressures taken. They both are concerned when Mr. T s blood pressure is found to be 170/ 85, and his grandson's is 120/60. Your best advice to them should be:*

    a. Not to be alarmed as this is not abnormal.
    b. Not to be alarmed, but to have their physician evaluate the grandfather's blood pressure.
    c. Suggest that Mr. T get his blood pressure treated.
    d. Privately tell the grandson to have Mr. T visit his physician.

As mentioned in question 19, more rigid vessels and narrower lumen can cause a rise in blood pressure with age, so it would not be surprising to find that Mr. T has a higher blood pressure than his grandson. The excitement at having his blood pressure evaluated could influence an elevation, as well. Although there is no cause for immediate alarm, it could be useful for Mr. T to visit his physician for reevaluation of his blood pressure since it did exceed 140/90, the World Health Organization's level for defining hypertension (Knudsen 1984, 224). It may be that this is an acceptable level for Mr. T, but it is wise to obtain medical evaluation. Since gerontological nurses are to include the client in the care process, it would not be appropriate to exclude Mr. T from the discussion by privately talking with the grandson.

    When evaluating blood pressure, it is important to assess the total person. Higher blood pressures may be necessary to compensate for circulatory problems; lowering a blood pressure to a level that looks acceptable on paper is meaningless if function is jeopardized. For example, on antihypertensive therapy Mr. T's blood pressure could drop to 110/60 and cause him to be confused and dizzy because of insufficient cerebral circulation. A level that maximizes function while minimizing risks should be maintained.

Respiratory Changes

22. *A nursing student wants to initiate breathing exercises for a nursing home resident to aid in improving respirations, and asks your advice. You know that based on the elderly's usual respiratory changes, it would be best to:*

   a. Have an expiration to inspiration ratio of 3:1
   b. Focus more on inspirations
   c. Avoid deep respirations
   d. Avoid these exercises altogether

The nursing student's idea to initiate breathing exercises is a sound one, particularly when all the factors that can reduce respiratory activity are considered. Lung expansion can be reduced because of weaker thoracic and diaphragm muscles, increased rigidity of the rib cage, and the increased anterior-posterior chest diameter that often accompanies advanced age. The alveoli are fewer in number and stretched. Decreased lung expansion affects expiration more than inspiration, thereby increasing residual volume. A debilitated or less mobile individual, as may be the case of a nursing home resident, would have even greater problems with effective respiration. Breathing exercises can benefit all older adults and be beneficial in preventing respiratory problems. Since expiration presents a greater problem, the exercises should focus on forced expiration: inhale deeply to the count of one and exhale to the count of three. The client should be instructed to pull in the abdomen upon expiration and push out while inhaling. The upper portion of the chest shouldn't move during these exercises; movement indicates shallow breathing.

Respiratory problems are the most common type of acute illness experienced by the elderly, and pneumonia and influenza rank as the fourth leading causes of death. Thus, aggressive attention to preventing respiratory illness is important. In addition to breathing exercises, measures such as good hydration and pneumonia and influenza vaccines are helpful. Subtle signs of respiratory infections should be noted, including changes in vital signs, mental status, and characteristics of sputum. Classic signs of penumonia may be absent in the elderly because of altered body pain sensations, decreased cough efficiency, and lower baseline body temperatures. Older adults should be advised to monitor "colds" carefully.

A cold that has not improved in a few weeks could be a more serious respiratory problem. Self-medication with over-the-counter cold remedies can mask symptoms and allow a serious condition to progress.

Gastrointestinal Changes

23. *Which is not associated with normal aging of the gastrointestinal tract?*

    a. Reduction in taste sensation
    b. Loss of teeth
    c. Decrease in gastric acid secretion
    d. Delayed emptying time of stomach

The gastrointestinal system is the source of many complaints by older persons, as most gerontological nurses are well aware. Food intolerance, indigestion, and constipation are often described. There are a multitude of changes that affect this system with age, including:

- atrophy of the taste buds (primarily affecting sensations for sweet and salty flavors)
- less saliva production
- decreased salivary ptyalin
- slower movement of food down the esophagus
- reduced stomach motility and emptying
- decreased hunger contractions
- less production of hydrochloric acid, pepsin, lipase, and pancreatic enzymes
- varying degrees of atrophy in intestines
- decreased peristalsis
- duller nerve impulses in lower bowel
- reduced liver size and storage capacity

It is no wonder that the elderly complain about this system's function.

The one item not present in this list of changes is that of tooth loss. Clearly, this notion is a myth, not a real outcome of normal aging. This may surprise many persons who work with the elderly, since it is rare to find an older adult with a full set of natural teeth. True, the majority of today's older population is edentulous, but that is not a normal consequence of aging. A history of poor diet, inadequate tooth care, and lack of access to good dentistry have resulted in the prevalence of dentures among the elderly. Better living standards, increased knowledge of good dental health practices, better access to dental care, and improved dentistry will influence future generations growing old with more of their natural teeth in place.

It should be emphasized that regular dental check-ups remain important in old age. Dentists can detect oral cancers, infections, and other problems that can seriously jeopardize the total well-being of the individual. Also, as tissue structure changes with age, dentures may need to be readjusted to assure proper fit.

24. *Mr. J tells you he is constipated. Your initial step would be to:*

    a. Administer a bulk-forming laxative
    b. Do a rectal exam
    c. Ask him why he believes he is constipated
    d. Ignore his comment, but monitor his bowel habits

Although the risk of constipation is higher with advanced age, and there are many factors that contribute to this problem, many older persons become unnecessarily concerned about bowel elimination because they fail to have a daily bowel movement. Straining to pass hard stool, infrequent bowel movement, and abdominal distention can mean constipation; the lack of a daily bowel movement alone does not. You would want to approach Mr. J's concern as you would any other nursing problem: by assessing first. Ask him about the frequency of his bowel movements, ease of defecation, and characteristics of stool. You may complete your assessment by performing a rectal exam, but your *initial* step would be to question him to gather additional data. Ignoring his problem wouldn't be appropriate, nor would administering a laxative without validating that constipation actually exists.

Genitourinary Changes

25. *Which description of bladder function would you believe to be a normal finding in late life?*

    a. Retention with anuria for as long as 24 hours
    b. Occasional incontinence
    c. Lack of sensation of need to void
    d. Frequency and nocturia

One annoying outcome of aging is the need to void more frequently due to weaker bladder muscles and a reduced bladder capacity (as low as 200 cc in some older persons). Most elderly individuals will have the need to void every few hours during the day, and at least once during the night. Although retention does become more prevalent with age, retention with anuria for as long as 24 hours would not be considered normal. The micturation reflex may be delayed in some older adults, but it is not normal for them to lack the sensation of the need to void.

Incontinence, occasional or not, is not to be considered normal. The occurrence of incontinence warrants a thorough evaluation. A variety of factors can be responsible for this problem, including urinary tract infection, prostatic enlargement, fecal impaction, obstruction of the bladder neck, medications, dehydration, neurologic disease, and altered mental status. Stress incontinence, whereby urine is lost during coughing or sneezing, is not uncommon in the elderly, particularly among older women. Exercises strengthen the pelvic floor muscles and surgical intervention may correct stress incontinence.

26. *During the home health nurse's visit, 72-year-old Mrs. M experiences an incontinent episode. Although Mrs. M has never complained of it before, upon questioning her, the nurse learns that Mrs. M has had incontinence for five to six months, but has never told any professional caring for her. You know that the most likely reason for Mrs. M's not sharing this problem is:*

    a. Altered mental status
    b. Lack of discomfort or distress over the problem
    c. Acceptance as a normal consequence of aging
    d. Desire to use this is an attention-getting measure

Many older adults (and even some health professionals) view incontinence as a normal outcome of aging, so they fail to bring this problem to anyone's attention, and this is the most likely reason for Mrs. M not sharing it. It is doubtful that she isn't affected by the problem, and there is no information in the question indicating any problem with Mrs. M's mental health.

27. *Which could be considered an abnormality of sexual function in the elderly?*

   a. Desire for masturbation
   b. Difficulty of penile penetration into the vagina
   c. Reduced frequency of intercourse
   d. Lack of reproductive ability in the male

Sexual interest and function do not disappear with age, although several significant sexual changes are evident. Older women will have some atrophy of the vulva; the vaginal epithelium becomes more fragile; and the vaginal canal is drier and more alkaline. Penile penetration can be more difficult for this reason. The cervix and uterus shrink, and the ovaries cease to function, causing a loss of reproductive function. The ability to enjoy sex and achieve orgasm are not reduced; in fact, some older females find new pleasure in sex once they needn't be concerned with pregnancy and have no children at home to disturb their intimacy. Men will find that it takes longer to achieve an erection, and more physical stimulation may be needed. It can be more difficult for an older man to regain an erection after an interruption or following ejaculation. The older male will have orgasms and ejaculate, although the ejaculation will probably be of a less forceful stream. Unlike the female, the male does not normally lose his reproductive abilities, which is why *d* is the correct answer.

Although the frequency of intercourse in late life may be less than in younger years, sexual patterns will not change significantly. Couples who enjoyed intercourse throughout their years together will continue to enjoy intimacy into late life; young persons who enjoyed oral sex or masturbation will not discontinue those activities at any magic age. Of course, persons who never derived much satisfaction from sex will be content to be sexually inactive. Keep in mind, however, that health problems, medications, lack of a partner, and concern about societal reaction can limit sexual activity in old age.

28. *The most significant obstacle preventing some older women from being sexually active is:*

    a. Lack of a partner
    b . Lack of knowledge
    c. Inability to have orgasms
    d. Vaginal atrophy

With the female to male ratio increasing with each advancing decade, it is little wonder that the most significant obstacle facing potentially sexually active older women is the lack of a partner. Earlier, it was stated that most older women are widowed, whereas most older men have living spouses. The majority of today's older females were raised to believe that sex outside of marriage is inappropriate; expectations from family and peers reinforce this belief. Without spouses, these women lack acceptable sexual partners.

Visual Changes

29. *Which is a visual change related to normal aging?*

    a. Color blindness
    b. Wider range of peripheral vision
    c. Farsightedness
    d. Blind spots in visual field

Sensory changes can profoundly affect the aging individual, and perhaps the most dramatic are those involving vision. Reduced accommodation and senile miosis are common, and presbyopia, the farsightedness accompanying aging, occurs in most people. This change actually begins to be noticed in middle age when most individuals find the need for corrective lenses.

Color blindness is not normal. There is a yellowing of the lens which causes low tone colors (blues, greens, violets) to become more difficult for older eyes to differentiate. Brighter colors can be seen more clearly.

There is a narrower, not wider, peripheral field seen by older eyes. To maximize visual capacity in the presence of this change, it is important to place objects within the visual field of the person; likewise, communication among elderly persons can be promoted by arranging seating in a circular fashion rather than in rows.

Retinal disease, such as macular degeneration and diabetic retinopathy, can be a cause for blind spots in the visual field. Although the incidence of this problem increases with age, it is not a visual change related to normal aging.

30. *Your 78-year-old nursing home resident complains that she doesn't like going outdoors on bright, sunny days because she can't see as well. You would recognize this to be associated with:*

    a. Presbyopia
    b. Glaucoma
    c. Early detached retina
    d. Cataracts

Cataracts develop at varying degrees in all aging persons. This opacity or clouding of the lens initially causes objects to appear blurred and can progress to severe visual impairment. One of the uncomfortable consequences of cataracts is that glare becomes more bothersome to the eyes. Fluorescent lighting, sunlight pouring through a window, and other forms of brightness that may not be noticed by younger eyes can cause significant annoyance to the elderly, reducing their visual capacity. Using indirect lighting and filtering bright light are beneficial measures for the person affected by cataracts.

Glaucoma ranks second to cataracts as a major eye problem affecting the elderly. This increase in intraocular pressure most typically occurs in the chronic form, accompanied by progressive reduction in visual field, tired eyes, headaches, misty vision, or seeing halos around lights. Acute glaucoma, a medical emergency, causes severe eye pain, nausea, vomiting, and blurred vision that will quickly progress to blindness, if not treated.

A detached retina, the forward displacement of the retina from the choroid, can appear gradually or suddenly. Persons with this problem will sense spots moving across their eyes, have blind areas of vision, feel there is a coating on their eyes, and see flashes of light.

31. *Which situation could result from a normal age-related change in vision?*

    a. Tripping while walking up the stairs
    b. Seeing halos around lights

    c. Not being able to see a dark wood door against a yellow
       wall
    d. Ignoring objects placed in the center of the visual field

An alteration in depth perception also accompanies the aging of the eyes. It becomes more difficult for the elderly to judge the height of curbs and stairs, which can lead to tripping and falls. Using a contrasting color where there are changes in levels and keeping such areas well lighted can help to reduce the risk of accidents.

Seeing halos around lights may be a result of glaucoma, a pathological condition which is not a normal outcome of aging; this symptom can also occur with digitalis toxicity. Rather than not being able to see a dark door against a yellow wall, the elderly probably would see the door more effectively, since color contrast is helpful in compensating for visual losses. Normally, peripheral vision would likely be reduced with age; thus, objects placed in the center of the visual field would be seen best.

Most people with visual limitations are over age 65. It is important that aging persons obtain regular eye examinations to detect visual problems early. The ability to see effectively can be crucial to the older adult's optimal physical, mental, and social health.

Hearing Loss

32. *The most effective approach to communicating with someone who has a high frequency hearing loss is to:*

    a. Have them use a hearing aid
    b. Speak in a loud, low-pitched voice
    c. Use a soft, whisper-like voice
    d. Teach them to use sign language

Presbycusis is the term used to describe the progressive hearing loss that occurs with age. High frequency sounds, particularly the *f, ph, s, sh,* and *ch* sounds are the first to be affected, followed by a loss of middle, and then low frequency sounds. This change is so subtle and gradual that many people fail to recognize that their hearing is impaired; they may blame their hearing problems on others' failure to speak clearly or loudly enough. Since high-pitched sounds present the most problem, communication can be enhanced by speaking loudly and clearly in a low-pitched voice. A screaming voice or a soft whisper will not be effective. Sign language will not be necessary for most persons affected by high frequency loss.

Hearing aids are seldom effective for high frequency losses. Even if a hearing aid is prescribed, adjustment can be difficult. Anyone with a hearing deficit should be advised to obtain a professional audiometric evaluation and not purchase a hearing aid unless it has been judged effective for the specific hearing loss present. Independently purchasing a hearing aid through a store or mail order catalogue can result in wasted dollars.

An often overlooked problem that can interfere with hearing is the impaction of cerumen. Cerumen hardens with age and can accumulate in the middle ear. Removing the wax by gentle irrigation can improve hearing in some persons. Clients should be advised not to use cotton tipped applicators to remove cerumen, as they can push it back and pack it harder. Also, no other foreign object (e.g., hairpins, toothpicks, rolled pieces of paper) should be placed in the ear.

Body Temperature

33. *Which statement most accurately explains why fever may appear atypically among the elderly?*

    a. Fever does not occur with infections.
    b. Normal body temperature may be lower.
    c. Temperature elevation can occur without cause.
    d. More often, hypothermia occurs with infection.

The response of the body to infection does not change with age; a temperature elevation occurs. Temperature elevation implies a problem and should not occur without a valid cause in old or young persons. The atypical feature of fever in the aged has to do with the fact that normal body temperature can be lower in older adults, thus an elevation would not present the high levels occurring in someone with a 98.6 degrees baseline temperature. For instance, a 2 degree elevation in a person with a normal temperature of 98.6 degrees would result in a temperature exceeding 100 degrees—a red flag triggering caregivers' attention. A temperature of 99 degrees may not cause similar concern and may even be ignored, although it could represent over a 2 degree elevation in an older person with a lower normal baseline temperature. Thus, fever may be defined at lower levels for older adults. It is important that body temperature be assessed while older adults are well so that normal baselines can be established and elevations recognized when they do occur.

Skin Changes

34. *A 74-year-old participant in a geriatric day care program tells you that she sponge-bathes daily and takes a tub bath only twice a week. Your best action would be to:*

    a. Schedule her for daily tub baths at the center
    b. Tell her to use alcohol for cleansing her skin during her daily sponge baths
    c. Do nothing
    d. Ask her why she won't bathe more frequently

This older client is demonstrating good judgment by her bathing practices. With age, the skin becomes more fragile and dry, and has less oil production and sweat gland activity. Unless a problem warrants differently (and there is nothing in the question indicating a problem exists) a complete bath every three to four days and a daily sponge bath should be sufficient for most older adults. More frequent bathing could rob the skin of its natural protection and result in excessive dryness and irritation. The drying effects of alcohol would discourage its use for sponge bathing.

35. *Sixty-four-year-old Mrs. F tells you she is concerned about the increasing number of "age spots" that have been appearing on her arms and hands. Your best response to her is:*

    a. "These are perfectly harmless"
    b. "You should have them biopsied"
    c. "Begin taking a vitamin supplement"
    d. "Blot them with bleach several times a day"

This pigmentation of the skin, commonly referred to as "age spots" or "liver spots," is due to a clustering of melanocytes that give the skin its color. They tend to occur on the body parts most exposed to the sun and are perfectly harmless. This skin pigmentation is not known to be associated with any pathology; thus, *b* and *c* are not appropriate responses. Although there are commercial preparations available to lighten these spots, it is not advisable to blot them several times daily with bleach because of the severe dryness to the skin that can result.

36. *A body change that seems to support the impact of radiation on the body's aging process is:*

    a. Melanocyte clustering
    b. Senile keratoses
    c. Osteoporosis
    d. Solar elastosis

Repeated exposure to sunlight and other sources of ultraviolet light can cause an aging or wrinkling of the skin known as solar elastosis. This loss of the skin's elasticity results from changes below the skin's surface, where the ultraviolet light causes collagen to be replaced by elastin. This change and the carcinogenic effects of overexposure to ultraviolet light support the practice of avoiding sunburns and limiting suntanning.

Sleep

37. *A friend expresses concern to you regarding her 75-year-old mother's insomnia, stating that her mother goes to bed at 9 p.m., but can be heard walking around the house and fixing snacks in the kitchen at 4 a.m. She asks your advice on how to help her mother. Your best response would be to tell her to:*

   a. Supply a protein-rich snack immediately before her mother goes to bed
   b. Obtain a comprehensive physical and mental examination of her mother
   c. Give her mother 2 aspirin and warm milk at bedtime
   d. Do nothing if her mother is not bothered

Older individuals do require more rest periods during the day, but they need less sleep at night. Five to seven hours of sleep are sufficient for most elderly persons. Since your friend's mother retires for bed at 9 p.m., she has achieved her full sleep requirement by 3 to 4 a.m. If the mother wishes to sleep later, she could try staying awake to a later hour, but if she is not bothered by this early awakening, there is no need to intervene. Slower digestive processes and higher risk of aspiration would make food intake immediately before bedtime an unsound measure; likewise, using a medication unnecessarily can create new problems.

Diet

38. *The diet of the older adult should consist of:*

   a. More calories of higher quality
   b. Double the vitamin and iron intake
   c. Fewer calories of higher nutritional value
   d. Higher amounts of protein, vitamins and minerals; no fats

Throughout the adult years, a gradual reduction in caloric intake is warranted, although those fewer calories need to represent a well-balanced diet of high nutritive value. The vitamin and mineral intake for older adults does not differ significantly from that of younger adults, unless a health problem requires supplementation. Fat intake is restricted to 30-35 percent of the total caloric intake, but remains essential to the diet in old age because of the essential fatty acids and fat-soluble vitamins it contributes.

Nursing and Geriatric Health Problems

Assessment

39. *The most important reason for nursing assessment of the older adult is:*

    a. To identify nursing problems
    b. To detect medical problems missed by the physician
    c. To fulfill regulatory requirements
    d. To determine level of care for reimbursement

Although the realities of practice settings and pressures for documentation sometimes cause nurses to forget the real purpose, nursing assessment aids in identifying nursing problems and in formulating nursing diagnoses. This is consistent with the Standards for Gerontological Nursing Practice and sound professional practice.

Hypothermia

40. *Which older person is at lowest risk for hypothermia?*

    a. A surgical patient in the recovery room
    b. A thin individual who never shivers
    c. A woman who shivers a lot
    d. A person who consumes a moderate amount of alcohol

A body temperature of 95 degrees F (35 degrees C) or below is considered hypothermia. In general, the elderly have a higher risk of developing this problem because of their reduced ability to adapt to temperature changes, decreased constriction of surface vessels in response to cold (making them less aware of being cold), and higher prevalence of being debilitated, immobile, or malnourished. The effects of anesthesia and the typically cool temperatures in operating rooms place older surgical patients at risk. Alcohol causes a greater loss of heat from the body and can contribute to hypothermia. Since shivering produces heat, the thin individual who doesn't shiver not only lacks natural insulation, but can't produce the emergency heat she needs. The woman who shivers a lot is in the best position to protect herself from hypothermia.

It is important to monitor elderly persons carefully for hypothermia. This requires the use of thermometers that register below 95 degrees and the recognition of clues, such as a change in mental status, shivering, and the absence of complaints about being cold. Protection from cold temperatures is crucial; extremities, in particular, must be kept warm. Indoor environmental temperatures must be considered, also, since room temperatures below 70 degrees can be too cool for the elderly. Clients who are immobile or taking a CNS depressant need special observation and measures to increase their circulation. Slow rewarming of the body (1 degree per hour) is used to treat hypothermia. The mortality rate from this problem is high.

Cardiovascular Problems

41. *Which statement is true regarding myocardial infarctions in the elderly?*
   a. **Chest pain may not always occur.**
   b. They seldom occur in the absence of a history of cardiac disease.
   c. Few elderly survive them.
   d. Oxygen is not used in the treatment.

Altered pain sensations can cause a distortion in the presentation of myocardial infarction in the aged. The crushing chest pain may be absent; instead, a fluttering or feeling mistaken for indigestion may occur. A change in mental status may be the first indication of the problem, accompanied by moist, pale skin, a low-grade fever, drop in blood pressure, dyspnea, and a pulse that changes in either direction. Laboratory findings assist in confirming the diagnosis and can include serum glutamic oxalacetic transaminase (SGOT), creatinine phosphokinase (CPK), lactic dehydrogenase (LDH), elevated white blood cell count, and erythrocyte sedimentation rate. Characteristic EKG changes associated with a myocardial infarction may not occur until some tissue necrosis has occurred (approximately 12-24 hours). Most elderly do survive a heart attack and need education and support as they adjust their lifestyles to promote cardiovascular health.

Oxygen is used in the treatment of myocardial infarction and requires careful monitoring. The reduced ability to excrete carbon dioxide, creates a risk of carbon dioxide narcosis; thus, high levels of oxygen intake are usually contraindicated. Cyanosis may not occur with hypoxia, particularly if the individual is anemic (a common problem in the elderly); so other signs must be observed.

Most myocardial infarctions are caused by ischemic heart disease, although they can occur in the absence of any previous cardiac disease.

42. *The nursing assistant summons your help, and you find her trying to support an elderly patient who has fallen to the floor in a semiconscious state. This patient has a history of coronary artery disease, diabetes, and osteoporosis. The nursing assistant states that nothing unusual happened—the patient was straining to have a bowel movement and then suddenly collapsed. You could suspect this episode to be a result of:*

    a. Spontaneous fracture
    b. Hyperglycemic reaction
    c. The Valsalva maneuver
    d. Bowel obstruction

Although the patient is at risk for any of the problems listed in the possible answers, the circumstances involved would point to the Valsalva maneuver as being responsible. With the Valsalva maneuver, there is vagal stimulation and bradycardia. Insufficient cerebral circulation may have been responsible for the patient's altered level of consciousness.

43. *Which would you not expect to be true of a stasis ulcer in older adults?*

    a. They are at greater risk of developing in diabetic or obese persons.
    b. The affected extremity will be cooler than the one without the ulcer.
    c. Most occur near the ankle.
    d. Three-fourths of them eventually make amputation necessary.

Stasis ulcers of the legs are associated with venous or arterial insufficiency, hypertension, fungal infections, and neurologic and metabolic disorders; thus, diabetic and obese persons would be among the high risk groups. Most of these ulcers do occur near the ankle, and they vary in size. Arterial ischemic ulcers will be more painful than venous ones. The affected leg will be edematous, cool to the touch, and red, becoming pale when elevated. Treatment goals are to control infection and improve circulation in the lower extremity. Although most of these ulcers heal, there is a risk of amputation, so prevention and careful monitoring are important.

Respiratory Problems

44. *Your 78-year-old patient in respiratory distress is prescribed nasal oxygen at 3 liters. A nursing student asks you why a lower level than that normally prescribed is being used when this patient is having trouble breathing. Your accurate response is:*

   a. Fewer cells in the older body place a lower demand for oxygen
   b. Higher levels of infusion irritate the fragile tissue along the nasal passage
   c. The elderly are started on small doses, which are gradually increased
   d. A higher infusion could depress respirations and lead to carbon dioxide build-up

As discussed earlier, the reduced ability of the lungs to expel carbon dioxide contributes to a carbon dioxide accumulation. Increasing oxygen infusion raises the blood oxygen level and sends a message to the brain to decrease respirations. At the same time, respirations are reduced and less carbon dioxide is eliminated, high levels of oxygen would continue to be pumped in and additional carbon dioxide produced. The result is carbon dioxide narcosis, which could be fatal.

45. *A true statement regarding tuberculosis in the elderly is:*

   a. It is usually a reactivation of an earlier infection
   b. Increased immunity to the disease is developed with age

    c. Tuberculin skin tests are not effective in older persons
    d. It becomes less of a problem in old age

Although the frail state of some elderly individuals increases their risk of contracting TB, most cases are reactivations of earlier infections. Diagnosis can be delayed because the symptoms can be confused with other geriatric disorders (e.g., anorexia, weight loss, fatigue), or appear atypically (e.g., no night sweats due to decreased diaphoresis). The tuberculin skin test and other diagnostic measures employed with younger adults would be used with the elderly. Tuberculosis does occur with greater incidence with advanced age; thus, regular screening of high-risk individuals can be beneficial.

46. *Persons with a ruddy, pink complexion who are labelled "pink puffers" can be best believed to possess which of these diseases?*

    a. Pulmonary edema
    b. Chronic bronchitis
    c. Emphysema
    d. Pneumonia

The ruddy, pink complexion present in many persons with emphysema results from hypoxia associated with an elevated blood carbon dioxide level. Persons with emphysema will have dyspnea, cough, anorexia, weight loss, weakness, and a barrel chest from an increased anterior-posterior chest diameter. Good hydration and nutrition, maintenance of a patent airway, prevention of complications, and instruction in breathing exercises are essential components of the care plan.

47. *In performing postural drainage for an older person, you would do all of the following except:*

    a. Administer the prescribed aerosal medication prior to the postural drainage
    b. Perform the procedure before meals
    c. Use more forceful chest pounding to loosen secretions
    d. Change positions slowly

The basic procedure for postural drainage is similar for the older client; however, the more brittle and fragile bones of the elderly warrant more gentle pounding. It is also important to remember to have the client change positions slowly to prevent dizziness from blood pressure changes.

Gastrointestinal Problems

48. *Your 66-year-old neighbor tells you he has just been diagnosed as having a hiatal hernia and asks you how he can manage this problem. You would be correct in recommending that he:*

   a. Eat several, smaller meals throughout the day, rather than the three large ones he currently eats
   b. Consume a large dairy product snack within a half-hour before retiring to bed
   c. Use an antacid every four hours
   d. Sleep in a perfectly flat position

Hiatal hernias increase in incidence with age and can create the uncomfortable symptoms of heartburn, belching, regurgitation, and vomiting. The symptoms worsen when the client is in a recumbent position, especially if there has been recent food intake; thus, it would not be wise to suggest that a large snack be consumed before going to bed. Antacids may be part of the treatment plan, but it is not within the realm of nursing practice to prescribe medications.

Replacing three large meals with several smaller ones throughout the day can assist in reducing the volume of food in the stomach at one time and facilitating digestion. (This is actually a sound suggestion for older adults without hiatal hernias.)

49. *Your 82-year-old patient complains of abdominal discomfort and diarrhea. In examining her, you note that she has abdominal fullness, is lethargic, and has fecal matter on her nightgown; her appetite has been poor for several days. What would be the wisest course of action you could take?*

   a. Perform a rectal examination
   b. Collect a stool specimen for culture
   c. Obtain an order for an antidiarrheal drug
   d. Keep her NPO for the next 24 hours until the physician can examine her tomorrow

Since your patient has described her symptoms, and you have examined her abdomen and general condition, the next action in collecting your full database would be to perform a rectal examination. A stool specimen may not be necessary and, while waiting for results, correction of the problem could be delayed. If this patient's problem is fecal impaction, as the symptoms would indicate, an antidiarrheal drug will do her more harm than good. Unnecessary fluid restriction could risk dehydrating this patient. Through a rectal exam, a fecal mass may be palpated, and what seemed to be diarrhea may actually be fecal matter that has oozed around the impaction.

Diabetes

50. *Dr. J tells you not to bother testing the urine of his elderly diabetic patient because he prefers having her blood glucose evaluated. Why would he be selecting blood tests over urine samples?*

   a. Older persons can be hyperglycemic without spilling glucose into their urines.
   b. Clinitest and other urine testing methods are not sensitive to the elderly's urine.
   c. Glucose in the blood is more stable than glucose in the urine.
   d. There is no rationale for his preference.

Kidney changes with age can result in a higher renal threshold for glucose; consequently, a significant increase in blood glucose may occur before there is glycosuria. Urine testing alone would show a false-negative; therefore, blood glucose screening would be more reliable.

51. *Which statement is not true regarding glucose tolerance testing in older adults?*

   a. Age-related gradients are used in interpreting the test.
   b. Large doses of salicylates can reduce blood glucose and alter results.
   c. Older adults can have a normal fasting blood glucose but be hyperglycemic after carbohydrate intake.
   d. Carbohydrates are eliminated from the diet several days before testing.

The diagnosis of diabetes in the elderly is not an easy task. In addition to urine samples being unreliable, older persons can have normal fasting blood glucose levels while experiencing significant hyperglycemia after meals. The glucose tolerance test is the most reliable diagnostic measure. There are several factors that can alter the results of glucose tolerance tests. For instance, estrogen, furosemide, and certain diuretics can decrease glucose tolerance, while propranolol, and high doses of salicylates can lower blood glucose. Stress, illness, and poor dietary intake can cause glucose intolerance and can also affect results. It is recommended that at least 150 grams of carbohydrate be ingested for several days prior to testing. Higher blood glucose levels normally occur with advanced age; therefore, age-adjusted values must be used in interpreting glucose tolerance tests in the elderly. Several tests may be necessary to confirm a diagnosis.

Hypoglycemia is a much greater threat to older persons than hyperglycemia is. It is easy for hypoglycemia to be missed in the elderly, since the classic signs are altered; a change in mental status may be the first clue of the problem. Arrhythmias, myocardial infarction, strokes, and death can result from uncorrected hypoglycemia, so early detection and correction are crucial.

Genitourinary Problems

52. *Your 69-year-old patient asks to be taken to the bathroom every 15 minutes. Your best reaction would be:*

   a. Tell her she needn't toilet so frequently, as her bladder can actually hold more urine
   b. Ask her why she needs to toilet so frequently and if she voids each time she toilets
   c. Toilet her, recognizing this as a normal consequence of aging
   d. Toilet her every two hours and have her wear an adult diaper

Rather than take any action, you need to assess if there is anything unusual about this patient's voiding pattern by obtaining more data. Perhaps she is experiencing urinary frequency due to a urinary tract infection and really does need to void every 15 minutes; maybe she had an episode of incontinence and wants to toilet frequently to avoid an accident. Telling her that she needn't void so often won't stop her from needing to if a valid problem exists. Although frequency is common among the elderly, voiding every 15 minutes would hardly be considered a normal consequence of aging. Diapering her in this situation not only carries psychological implications, but it avoids addressing the underlying cause for her increased toileting.

53. *The laboratory indicates that a slight elevation in bacteria was found in Mrs. D's urine. You are surprised because she has shown no signs indicating a urinary tract infection. Mrs. D's physician is informed and states that he chooses not to treat her at this time, but will push fluids and monitor her. The reason for the physician's nontreatment can best be explained by:*

    a. Prescribing antibiotics could encourage a new strain of bacteria to emerge
    b. Physicians generally lack interest in older patients
    c. Antibiotics are not effective in treating urinary tract infections in the elderly
    d. A majority of older people have some degree of urinary tract infection

In addition to the resistance to the antibiotic that could develop, Mrs. D could develop a variety of complications from the drug. If she shows no other signs of infection, it would be best to observe her closely, force fluids, and promote acidic urine.

54. *Which is an accurate statement regarding prostatic hypertrophy in old age?*

    a. Black males have twice the rate of white males
    b. Most prostatic surgeries do not cause impotency
    c. Incontinence is a primary sign
    d. Most cases develop into malignancies

This not uncommon problem does have a higher incidence among white males. Symptoms develop subtly and gradually, and include hesitancy, reduced stream of urine flow, frequency, nocturia, and dribbling. Diagnosis is confirmed through palpation of the enlarged gland during rectal examination, cystourethroscopy, and evaluation of blood, urine, and renal tests. Most cases can be managed medically, and those that do require surgery most often involve a transurethral resection, which does not cause impotency. Although most prostatic enlargement is benign, a minority of men do develop malignancies; therefore, periodic evaluation is essential.

55. *"Hot flashes" in aging women:*

   a. Result from lowered estrogen levels
   b. Are associated with cardiovascular changes having nothing to do with the reproductive system
   c. Are of greater prevalence among women who have had multiple pregnancies
   d. Have no physiological basis

Hot flashes are not a myth or a false claim; they result from changes in the subcutaneous capillaries that occur from lowered estrogen levels. They are the most distressful symptom experienced during the climacteric.

56. *A nurse friend who is employed in a gynecologist's practice tells you that she has recently seen several older women in the office being treated for vaginitis and asks you if there is any special reason for this. Your most accurate response would be:*

   a. The more alkaline secretions of the older female's vagina place her at higher risk of infection
   b. In older women, this is a common precancerous sign
   c. This is usually associated with estrogen replacement therapy
   d. This is an extremely rare occurrence

Thinner, more alkaline vaginal secretions, and a more delicate, atrophic vaginal mucosa set the stage for senile vaginitis. Although symptoms of vaginitis are similar for young and old women, some older women do not recognize that this infection can likewise occur in the elderly, and they may thus not seek evaluation. Women, with altered mental status or other impairments may be unable to express their symptoms; thus, special nursing observation is warranted.

Older women need to be educated on the importance of regular gynecological examinations. Some older women may have never used a gynecologist, while others may believe there is no need for a gynecological examination after childbearing years; clarification and reinforcement of the continued importance of these exams are necessary. Gynecological examination of institutionalized females should be scheduled regularly, also.

Neurological Problems

57. Mrs. S has a history of glaucoma. Which sign would indicate that Mrs. S is experiencing an increase in her intraocular pressure?

    a. Cloudy lens
    b. Loss of color vision
    c. Absence of tearing
    d. Dull headaches

An obstruction of the anterior chamber angle causes the increased intraocular pressure associated with glaucoma. The rise in intraocular pressure is accompanied by edema of the ciliary body and pupil dilation, resulting in a blurring of vision that can progress to blindness if untreated. Seeing a halo around lights, tearing of the involved eye, eye pain, nausea, and vomiting are experienced, as are dull, vague headaches. Tonometry is needed to evaluate the intraocular pressure.

58. Which of the following would most likely precipitate a transient ischemic attack in a person with a history of this problem?

    a. Quickly rising from a lying to a standing position
    b. Administration of aspirin on a regular basis
    c. Reduction in activity level
    d. Rapid change in weather conditions

A transient ischemic attack (TIA) can result from anything that reduces cerebral circulation, such as quickly rising to a standing position, "nodding off" while in a sitting position (which causes flexion or extension of the head and neck), smoking, and medications having a hypotensive effect. Symptoms last minutes to hours and include blackout, falling, amnesia, speech impairment, loss of vision (usually unilateral), diplopia, motor weakness, reduced sensations, and hemiparesis. Since a TIA is an important warning of possible cerebrovascular accident, prompt treatment is essential, as is the prevention of future TIAs. Daily doses of aspirin are being used in the treatment of males with TIAs with some success; anticoagulant therapy or surgical intervention can be employed, also. The hypotensive effects of quickly rising from a sitting position emphasize the need to instruct persons with this problem to rise slowly to a standing position.

Musculoskeletal Problems

59. *In examining a 68-year-old woman, you detect bony nodules on the joints of several of her fingers. You could suspect this to be associated with:*

   a. Rheumatoid arthritis
   b. Osteoporosis
   c. Osteoarthritis
   d. Paget's disease

The effects of joint degeneration become apparent in middle age and appear with increasing frequency with advanced age. This degenerative joint disease, osteoarthritis, primarily affects the weight-bearing joints, shoulders, and fingers. Joint pain and stiffness are present, which improve after the joint is used. Bony spurs, known as Heberden's nodes, commonly develop on the distal ends of the affected fingers, and crepitation may be heard with joint movement. Control of symptoms, exercise, and weight reduction are among the treatments employed.

Some older adults believe all forms of arthritis are similar and may not understand that their osteoarthritis is quite different from the severely disabling and deforming rheumatoid arthritis. Whereas osteoarthritis is limited to the joints, rheumatoid arthritis has systemic effects, such as a low-grade fever, anorexia, weight loss, anemia, and weakness. Nodules may be found over the bony prominences of the rheumatoid arthritis victim, but they are subcutaneous in origin; atrophy of the muscles on the affected extremity may occur. In addition to controlling symptoms, preventing deformities is an important measure.

60. *Which would not be a contributing factor in the development of gout?*

a. Underexcretion of uric acid
b. Overproduction of uric acid
c. Insulin therapy
d. Thiazide diuretic therapy

Gout results from the deposit of monosodium urate crystals in the joint spaces. This occurs as a result of the overproduction or underexcretion of uric acid; since thiazide diuretics can inhibit the excretion of uric acid, they can be a contributing factor. Although any joint can be affected, the great toe is the most common site for gout attacks. Several years of remission can occur between attacks.

61. *Next to the hip, a common site of fractures in the elderly is the:*

a. Wrist
b. Skull
c. Rib cage
d. Ankle

The high risk of accidents and osteoporosis contribute to fractures being a serious problem for older adults. The neck of the femur, wrist (Colles' fracture), and spinal column are the most common sites of fractures in the elderly. Because the bones do fracture more easily in old age, stresses that occur in normal daily activities (stepping off a high curb, twisting a tight lid off a jar, bumping against an object) can result in a broken bone. Whenever there is potential that a fracture may have occurred, the involved area should be immobilized and an X-ray obtained. In addition to treatment of the fracture and control of symptoms, early rehabilitation is important in promoting optimal recovery and independence.

62. *A patient on your unit returns from physical therapy with a cane to assist in his ambulation. You would know that the correct use of this cane consists of positioning it on:*

a. The affected side and advancing it with the affected leg
b. The affected side and advancing it with the unaffected leg
c. The unaffected side and advancing it with the affected leg
d. The unaffected side and advancing it with the unaffected leg

Canes are used to provide stability, conserve energy, relieve pressure on weight-bearing joints, and compensate for impaired function. The proper fit of the cane is for the handle to be level with the greater trochanter, with the client's elbow flexed approximately 30 degrees. Placing the cane on the unaffected side and advancing it with the affected side provides the greatest support and stability.

63. *You are assisting a wheelchair-bound person who has right-sided weakness in returning to bed. Your appropriate positioning of the wheelchair is to place it so that:*

   a. The patient's right side is next to the bed
   b. The patient's left side is next to the bed
   c. The chair is facing the bed, approximately two feet away
   d. The chair is parallel to the foot of the bed

To provide maximum use of this client's stronger side, it would be wise to place the client's left side closest to the bed so that he or she can lift and pivot more effectively. Wheelchairs should be fitted individually, based on the client's height, weight, and functional abilities.

Mental Health and Illness

Assessment

64. *During the mental status examination portion of the assessment, you request the client to do all of the items described in a-d below. Which one is the best test of the client's judgment?*

   a. Pick up the paper, fold it in half, and hand it to me
   b. Place the pegs in the holes as quickly as you can
   c. Explain what is meant by "A bird in the hand is worth two in the bush"
   d. Count backwards from 100 by 7's

Most tests of cognitive function include questions pertaining to the client's:

• orientation: person, place, time

- ability to follow a three-stage command, as described in response *a*
- judgment, in which problem-solving and reasoning capabilities are explored, exemplified by response *c*
- memory: short- and long-term
- calculation, such as that shown in response *d*

Response *b* tests psychomotor speed more than cognitive function and would be limited in the insight it would yield into mental status. General mood, behavior, body language, level of consciousness, perceptions, and symptoms shared by the client are, of course, integral components of the mental status examination.

Mental status assessment must be put in the perspective of the client's present situation. A variety of physical problems can alter mental status; thus, confusion or other signs of mental impairment may require medical rather than psychiatric intervention. Medications can cause changes in mental status, as can stressful situations (such as admission to a hospital). It must be remembered that the mental status evaluation may reflect only a snapshot of the client's status at that particular time; repeated assessments may be required to obtain a more accurate understanding of the client's general mental health.

65. *Seventy-three-year-old Mrs. R comes to the clinic accompanied by her daughter. The daughter states that Mrs. R has seemed confused lately. Your best response is to:*

    a. Send Mrs. R for a complete physical examination
    b. Interview Mrs. R and her daughter to learn more about her possible confusion
    c. Recognize this as the daughter's anxiety and reassure her that there is probably nothing wrong
    d. Arrange for a home visit by the mental health nurse

Comprehensive data must be collected on clients before any action is taken. Response *a* implies that there is a problem requiring evaluation, an unknown fact under the circumstances. It isn't known if the daughter is anxious, so response *c* is making a false assumption. Response *d* may be unnecessary and a waste of resources. By interviewing Mrs. R and her daughter, the nurse can explore the symptoms and all factors can be considered, so that specific, appropriate plans can be developed.

Depression

66. *With which condition can depression sometimes be easily mistaken?*

    a. Anxiety
    b. Alcoholism
    c. Delirium
    d. Dementia

    Depression increases with age and is the most commonly presented psychiatric problem of the elderly. In addition to the sad emotional tone, depressed persons may display anorexia, weight loss, fatigue, insomnia, constipation, and a lack of interest in self-care. The physical consequences of these behaviors can lead to health problems which are manifested intially through confusion and dullness. Although many of the manifestations of depression mimic those of dementia, there is not a decline in intellectual abilities. Differential diagnosis is important and can be aided by careful nursing observation. Treatment of depression is beneficial in improving the quality of life and self-care capacity.

67. *Seventy-year-old Mr. O is the husband of one of your nursing home residents. His wife has been institutionalized for eight years and is in stable condition. Mr. O has maintained the family home during that time, although he has barely met his expenses. Last month he sold his car because of a significant rise in his insurance. Mr. O's daughter drives him to the facility for visits now, and during one of the visits she tells you that her father hasn't been himself lately: he is moping around, not eating his favorite foods that she prepares for him, losing interest in his appearance, and is generally, acting depressed. If Mr. O is depressed, it would most likely be associated with:*

    a. His wife's condition
    b. Limited finances
    c. Household burdens
    d. Ceasing to drive

Although all of the responses are factors challenging Mr. O's mental health, he has been managing *a, b,* and *c* for the years that his wife has been institutionalized. Most probably, the factor responsible for his new display of depression is the most recent change or loss he experienced: ceasing to drive. This loss may threaten his independence, limit his ability to visit his wife, and be one more stress than he is able to manage.

68. *Which group has the highest rate of suicide?*
    a. White males over age 75
    b. Late stage Alzheimer's victims
    c. Black males ages 65-75
    d. White widows over age 70

One-quarter of all suicides in this country are committed by persons over age 65, most of whom are older white males. Although persons with dementia are a high risk group for suicides, it is usually in the early stages, when the loss of intellectual function is realized and the ability to execute a plan is possible, that suicide is most likely. All threats of suicide from older adults should be taken seriously.

Dementia

69. *Mr. C is visiting the mental health clinic for assessment of his dementia. Halfway through the routine interview he becomes hostile and refuses to answer any more questions. Your best action is to:*
    a. Discontinue the interview
    b. Ignore his reaction and proceed
    c. Ask him if he is feeling insulted or embarrassed by the questions being asked
    d. Explain to him that this information will help in planning individualized care for him

Mr. C is demonstrating a "catastrophic reaction" in which he is feeling overwhelmed with the situation at hand. This is not uncommon in persons with dementia who have a limited capacity to manage situations. Ignoring the reaction and continuing with the interview will increase his stresses and worsen the situation. Response *c* implies that Mr. C has insight into his behavior and ignores the real cause of the reaction. The importance of the interview for individualizing his care will mean little to Mr. C, who is primarily interested in retreating from a situation he can't manage. It will be more effective to discontinue the interview and attempt to collect the data at another time. To prevent catastrophic reactions, it is useful to break tasks into smaller pieces that the client can manage and avoid placing the client in situations known to exceed his or her intellectual capabilities.

70. *One of the nursing home residents with mutli-infarct dementia has asked for the time several times in the past hour. On her next request, your best response would be to:*

   a. Tell her the time
   b. Tell her you have told her the time and to try to remember what you told her
   c. Ask her why she continues asking the same question
   d. Tell her she is annoying others by asking for the time

It is reasonable to believe that this patient does not have the cognitive ability to remember information given to her, thus responses *b, c,* and *d* are not appropriate. If this lady's abilities permit, it could be useful to supply her with a clock or watch of her own.

This type of behavior can be frustrating to caregivers who don't understand that it is part of the patient's illness. Caregiver education and support are important in helping them cope with the demands of being cognitively impaired.

71. *The most important environmental factor in aiding the function of Alzheimer's victims is:*

   a. Variety
   b. Unrestricted wandering
   c. High stimulation
   d. Consistency

A simple, stable environment can enhance the function of someone with impaired cognitive function. The stress of variety and high stimulation can overwhelm Alzheimer's victims and make them less functional. Unrestricted wandering can result in serious safety risks for these individuals who lack adequate judgment to protect themselves. Placement of objects in the same location at all times, adhering to routines, and assigning the same caregivers to these patients are beneficial measures.

Grief

72. *You visit Mrs. B three weeks after her husband's death. Her sister, widowed five years ago, is with her and you find them both crying. The sister tells you that she can sympathize with Mrs. B because she too was married almost 50 years and still thinks about her husband all the time; she claims she is unable to sleep through the night without crying over his death. Mrs. B shakes her head in agreement and says, "Yes, that is how it is with me." Your best response to Mrs. B would be:*

    a. It is normal to feel this way so soon after your husband's death. In time, these feelings will lessen.
    b. You shouldn't keep grieving your loss, but get on with your own life.
    c. You'd be better off giving yourself time alone and not listening to other widows.
    d. Although the pain you are feeling will be a constant part of your life, you must try to find happiness.

Within the first few days following a death, it is normal for the surviving loved ones to be in a state of shock whereby they feel numb to the world around them. This is followed by the reality of the loss setting in, and profound grief. During the latter stage, survivors may feel empty, depressed, angry, and guilty. Support from friends, family, clergy, and professionals can aid survivors in expressing and resolving their feelings. They need to know that their feelings and behaviors are accepted as normal manifestations of the grieving process. It is also important to emphasize that the pain they may now be feeling will subside in time. Normally, within one year following the death, the grieving process should be completed. Response *b* ignores the necessary expression of grief that must occur so soon after Mr. B's death, and that advice is hardly therapeutic. Since other widows can provide a new network of support and friendship for Mrs. B, *c* would not be an appropriate comment. To imply that the profound grief Mrs. B is feeling so soon after her husband's death will be a constant part of her life could be overwhelming to her, and is thus an incorrect response.

73. *In the aforementioned situation, you recognize Mrs. B's sister's grief to be:*

    a. Unresolved and abnormal
    b. A normal reaction to a long, happy marriage that has ended
    c. An attention-getting mechanism
    d. A compensation for the poor relationship she had with her husband while he was alive

If after five years of widowhood, the sister continues to grieve actively and experience disruption to her life, unresolved grief may be present. You would want to assess the sister to help determine the reason for this continued grief and how it is affecting her life. Therapeutic intervention, such as professional counselling, may be warranted.

74. *Widowed Mr. W spends most of his day in activities related to his pet dog. He takes the dog for long walks, cooks a full dinner that the dog gets a portion of, and is constantly writing his children anecdotes about the dog's latest pranks. Your best reaction to the situation would be to:*

    a. Counsel Mr. W to focus the same attention on a human being rather than a dog
    b. Obtain a mental status evaluation
    c. Contact his children to discuss ways to expand his social world
    d. Do nothing

Pets play an important and therapeutic role in the lives of many older persons. They can be the motivation for the elderly to awaken in the morning, eat, and exercise. In addition to the pleasure derived from interacting with a pet, there may be greater opportunities for the individual to interact with other humans, using the pet as the "conversation piece." Pets can also serve as a source of protection by warning their owners of intruders, fires, and other unusual circumstances. There is no indication that Mr. W is having any problems related to having a pet, so there is no need to intervene.

It should be remembered that the loss of a pet can cause profound grief for the elderly, leading to possible health threats. Clients' grief over the loss of a pet should be facilitated and not belittled. Every assessment should include a review of pets and the role they play in the client's life.

Geropharmacology

General Principles

75. *A general rule of thumb regarding geriatric pharmacology is:*
   a. Except for cardiac drugs, all medications should be prescribed in greater amounts
   b. Drugs are less effective in late life
   c. Most drugs do more harm than good
   d. Lower doses of most medications should be used

With fewer functioning nephrons, a reduction in glomerular filtration rate, and less circulation through the kidneys, it takes longer for drugs to be eliminated. The longer period in which the drugs are present in the bloodstream can result in their accumulating to toxic levels, causing adverse reactions. To compensate for this, most medications are prescribed in lower dosages.

Drug therapy in late life becomes quite complicated and risky. Numerous health problems among the elderly tend to encourage the use of more drugs, and with each additional drug they take, the risk of complications increases significantly. Lack of knowledge can lead to dangerous self-medication by the elderly; visual deficits can cause self-administration errors. Drug absorption can be impaired by changes in gastric acid secretion, metabolism, body temperature, circulation, and state of hydration. Signs of adverse reactions can appear differently (confusion is often a sign presented in the elderly), thereby delaying the recognition of a problem. This is not to imply that drugs should not be used with the elderly; pharmacologic advances have given many persons a longer and more functional life. Rather, drugs need to be used and monitored more carefully in older adults. Whenever a drug is prescribed, the nurse needs to ask if:

- the drug is truly necessary
- a nonpharmacologic method can be substituted
- the dosage is age-adjusted
- the drug will interact with other drugs or food

- special precautions or actions must be employed

Periodic reevaluation of the drug's continued need and effectiveness is important, also.

Aspirin

76. *One problem with using acetaminophen in the management of arthritis is:*

   a. It lacks an anti-inflammatory effect
   b. A tolerance can develop
   c. It is not an effective analgesic in the elderly
   d. It can exacerbate joint pain as a potential side effect

Although acetaminophen is an effective analgesic and can relieve arthritic pain as well as aspirin can, it has no impact on the inflammation that accompanies arthritis. Aspirin, because of its effectiveness and relatively low cost, is a widely used drug among the elderly. It usually reaches its peak blood level within one to two hours. Gastric irritation is a common side effect of aspirin; poor nutritional status and signs of gastric ulcer formation should be observed. When reduction of inflammation is not necessary, acetaminophen can be substituted for aspirin to relieve gastric problems. Persons with a history of asthma or COPD can develop wheezing or bronchospasm as a reaction to aspirin therapy; thus, the relationship of respiratory symptoms to aspirin therapy must be considered. Higher blood levels of aspirin can result from a more acidic urine (this causes a greater tubular reabsorption of the drug), thereby discouraging the administration of high doses of ascorbic acid when aspirin is being taken.

Aspirin's effects can be decreased by antacids, phenobarbital, propranolol, and reserpine. Aspirin can increase the effects of oral anticoagulants, oral hypoglycemics, penicillin, and phenytoin. Indications of salicylate toxicity should be noted and include dizziness, tinnitus, hearing loss, vomiting, fever, convulsions, burning sensation in oral cavity, and confusion.

Digoxin

77. *Mr. R tells you he has been taking his digoxin with an antacid to prevent heartburn. You recognize that:*

a. This is a sound practice
b. The effects of digoxin can be increased
c. **The effects of digoxin can be decreased**
d. There will be no positive or negative effects from the antacid

Digoxin is alleged to be the fourth most commonly prescribed medication in this country. It reaches its peak within four to six hours and has a biological half-life (the amount of time it takes for one-half of the dose to be eliminated from the body) of 36 hours. Digitalis toxicity is a serious threat and is displayed by altered mental status, impaired color vision, blurred vision, seeing halos around dark objects, diplopia, dizziness, headaches, restlessness, muscle weakness and pain, ataxia, seizures, neuralgias, anorexia, nausea, vomiting, diarrhea, bradycardia, and congestive heart failure. A good potassium intake is essential during digoxin therapy as hypokalemia increases the risk of toxicity. Antacids, kaolin-pectin, laxatives, neomycin, phenobarbital, and phenylbutazone are among the drugs that can decrease digoxin's effects; the drug's effects can be increased by phenytoin and propranolol.

Miotics

78. *Mrs. U uses miotic eye drops for her glaucoma. She is scheduled for orthopedic surgery. You know that the eye drops should:*

a. Not be administered two days prior to surgery, but can be used immediately postoperatively
b. Not be used two days before or two days after surgery
c. **Be administered without interruption**
d. Be discontinued until her discharge from the hospital

Miotics, such as pilocarpine, aid in improving the outflow of aqueous humor, thereby helping to maintain a normal intraocular pressure. Sudden discontinuation of these drops can cause intraocular pressure to rise and serious retina damage to result. Thus, withholding the medication unnecessarily could be problematic. Since these cholinergic agents affect the eye and infrequently affect the entire system, it is unlikely that they will present a problem during orthopedic surgery. If a standard preoperative order to "discontinue all medications" is given, it would be advantageous to remind the physician of the ophthalmic drops and to clarify whether the order applies to them as well.

Laxatives

79. *Mr. H has been using mineral oil as a laxative daily over the past several months. Which of the following problems that he displays would be least likely to be associated with the use of mineral oil?*
   a. Respiratory infections
   b. Vitamin A and D deficiencies
   c. Diarrhea
   d. Fat particles in stool

The fact that oil-based laxatives have been used for generations and are relatively inexpensive makes them popular to some older adults. Although these "old standbys" seem benign, they can produce serious effects. The unpleasant taste of oil-based laxatives can make them difficult to ingest; the gagging and coughing that could accompany ingestion can lead to aspiration of the substance, resulting in lipoid pneumonia. Chronic use of mineral oil can interfere with the absorption of nutrients and vitamins, particularly the fat-soluble vitamins A, D, K, and E. Also, as with any laxative use, mineral oil can cause diarrhea and risk dehydrating the older individual. Because of the many risks associated with their use, oil-based laxatives are not recommended for use with the elderly.

Nitroglycerin

80. *Mr. T is using nitroglycerin ointment. In discussing his application of the ointment, he tells you that he uses the same site at all times (a hairless part of his arm), thoroughly removes all old ointment before the new application is made, and leaves the ointment on, untouched until the next application. The one change to Mr. T's procedure that you would recommend would be to:*
   a. Apply the ointment to the chest or abdomen rather than the arm
   b. Not wash off the former application
   c. Use different application sites each day
   d. Thoroughly remove the ointment four hours after application

Nitroglycerin is a vasodilator used to reduce the cardiac workload. Topical nitroglycerin can be applied to the chest, forearm, abdomen, or thigh. The site should be clean and dry, with as little hair as possible. The previous day's application should be cleansed before a new one is applied. Site rotation is recommended to prevent skin inflammation and sensitivity; it is useful to keep a record of sites used. The ointment should not be rubbed into the skin because this will increase the rate of absorption and decrease the sustained release of the medication. Covering the application site with plastic aids absorption by keeping the skin moist and prevents the ointment from being rubbed off. Nurses should be careful not to allow the ointment to come into contact with their skin, since it can be absorbed.

Since dizziness can occur following the administration of nitroglycerin, it is wise to have the client sit or lie down for a short period after application. Signs of adverse reactions should be noted. These include irregular and rapid pulse, hypotension, decreased respirations, blurred vision, muscle weakness, and confusion. The hypotensive effects of nitroglycerin can be increased by alcohol and propranolol. Tricyclic antidepressants and atropine-like drugs can become more potent when taken with nitroglycerin. Intraocular pressure can be increased by nitroglycerin; thus, close monitoring of a client with glaucoma is essential. Persons using nitroglycerin need regular follow-up to assess the medication's effectiveness and to identify possible adverse reactions.

Treatment of Gout

81. *Probenecid is effective in the treatment of gout by:*

   a. Inhibiting the kidney tubules' reabsorption of uric acid
   b. Inhibiting inflammation
   c. Depressing CNS function
   d. Relaxing muscle tissue

Since gout involves problems with the overproduction or underexcretion of uric acid, a drug attacking the underlying problem would be most helpful. Probenecid blocks the tubular reabsorption of urate, increasing urinary excretion of uric acid. It has no analgesic or antiinflammatory effects. When therapy is initiated, reactions must be observed closely: probenecid can exacerbate gout in the first few weeks of therapy, and concurrent administration of colchicine may be needed. Salicylates will have an antagonistic effect and should be avoided when probenecid is used. Probenecid can increase the hypoglycemic effect of chlorpropamide, and increase the effects of sulfonamides, rifampin, pantothenic acid, and indomethacin. Headaches, anorexia, nausea, vomiting, urinary frequency, dermatitis, pruritus, anemia, and formation of urate kidney stones are among the adverse reactions which must be noted.

Psychotropics

82. *Mr. L is demonstrating involuntary rhythmic movements of his tongue, face, and limbs. Which of the following medications he is receiving would be associated with this problem?*
   a. Digoxin
   b. Chloral hydrate
   c. Haloperidol
   d. Levodopa

   Antipsychotics, or tranquilizers, have been beneficial in controlling emotional disorders and in helping people live more functional lives. They do, however, carry the risk of many side effects. The rhythmic, involuntary movements that Mr. L displays are referred to as tardive dyskinesia, one of the adverse effects of antipsychotic therapy. He may show facial tics, blinking, lip smacking, tongue protrusion, and rolling movements; he may shrug his shoulders and rock his body; he may rotate his wrists and have a pill-rolling motion of his fingers. These extrapyramidal effects closely resemble Parkinson's disease and must be detected early to prevent permanent effects. Tardive dyskinesia is a greater risk to the elderly who have been using phenothiazines.
   Besides the fact that haloperidol is becoming less popular for use with the elderly, there is another potential problem with the administration of this drug to Mr. L. If you look at his drug list, you will see that one of the drugs being taken by Mr. L is levodopa, an antiparkinsonism drug. If Mr. L has parkinsonism, haloperidol administration is not recommended. This exemplifies a typical problem in prescribing patterns for the elderly: the total problems of the client may not be considered, or one practitioner may be unaware of the problems being managed by another practitioner. The nurse's role in coordinating care is to assure that such problems don't occur. This is an important concern in gerontological nursing.

Practice Issues

Service Delivery

83. *Which would you know to be a true statement regarding older nursing home residents?*

    a. There are the same number of older persons in psychiatric hospitals as in nursing homes.

    b. Most nursing home residents are widowed females.

    c. Only a small minority of nursing home residents have a mental illness.

    d. Most are private-pay patients.

In the United States, there are over 25,000 nursing homes, housing over 1.5 million individuals. Although less than 5 percent of the elderly reside in any type of institution at any given time, almost one-quarter will spend some time in a long-term care facility sometime before they die (U.S. Bureau of the Census 1986c). There are more than double the number of nursing home beds as hospital beds, a trend that will continue as hospital inpatient care declines and the number of elderly increase. Nursing homes can be skilled (meaning that the patient requires a higher level of care by professional staff) or intermediate (less intense care needs).

Most institutionalized persons are likely to be white, unmarried females who lived alone prior to their admissions. Since widowed females are prevalent among the geriatric population, it stands to reason that they would be more prevalent among the nursing home population. In addition to functional status, family resources play a significant role in preventing institutionalization.

Although rehabilitation and psychiatric hospitals, domicilliary facilities, and other types of institutional care are utilized by the elderly, more than three-quarters of those institutionalized reside in nursing homes. At least one-half of the nursing home population are supported by Medical Assistance or other forms of government support. (Even if a person enters a nursing home as a private-pay patient, it doesn't take long for the cost of care to dwindle life savings.) More than one-half of nursing home residents are estimated to possess some form of mental disorder; it is expected that this number will increase as deinstitutionalization from mental hospitals continues and persons with psychiatric disorders survive to later years (Johnson and Grant 1985, 38).

84. *The most significant factor believed to be responsible for the growth of nursing home beds is:*
   a. Increased number of elderly persons
   b. Decreased responsibility of families for care of the older relatives
   c. Passage of Medicare and Medical Assistance legislation in the 1960s
   d. Greater societal acceptance of this form of care

Efforts to provide institutional care to the aged and needy have existed since colonial times. Charitable organizations and governments provided a variety of "homes for the aged," "almshouses," and other facilities to provide basic shelter and personal care. Frequently, these facilities lacked adequate resources and had conditions which caused them to be viewed as an option of last resort. In 1935, Social Security was introduced, providing a means for older persons to purchase services independently; in response, small "homes" for the aged multiplied, often owned and operated by nurses (thus, the term "nursing home" grew). By 1960, there were over 9,000 nursing homes, with 290,000 residents; the number of facilities doubled, and the residents served tripled in the decade that followed. The factor promoting this growth was the 1965 passage of Medicare and Medical Assistance. The $500 million spent in 1960 on nursing home care grew to $4.7 billion by 1970, and now exceeds $30 billion. Although the percentage of older persons requiring institutional care is not expected to increase from its current level of 5 percent, that percentage will represent greater numbers of people; thus, the need for nursing home beds will continue. It is anticipated that the nursing home population will become an older, more frail, and more medically complicated one.

85. *In looking at future service needs of the older population, which would not be likely?*
   a. The elderly will have fewer health problems and service needs.
   b. More nursing home beds will be needed.
   c. Families will be providing more direct care for longer periods of time.

    d. The elderly will be paying for more services out of their own pockets.

More people are achieving old age in better states of health than ever before, but the fact that more are reaching the old-old years when the prevalence of disease and disability is higher, more health problems may be evident. Also, technologic and pharmacologic innovations have saved lives that would have not survived before, causing more people with health problems to reach old age. These individuals will present many service needs, as will the well elderly who are more knowledgeable and have higher expectations of the health care system.

As discussed in the previous question, more nursing home beds will be needed as the older population increases. Family members, particularly middle-aged women, will carry a greater responsibility for care of their elder relatives: more complicated care for longer periods of time than ever before. Current changes in the reimbursement system (e.g., limited lengths of stay, more stringent requirements for nursing home and home health care, greater Medicare copayments by the elderly) are a sample of the trend toward greater demands on the elderly for self-payment for care.

86. Which among the following is the most important factor in determining an older person's risk of institutionalization?

    a. Available family support
    b. Ability to pay
    c. Number of medical problems
    d. Desire of the individual

Having a spouse or other family members available as a support network and to serve as caregivers is the most significant factor influencing institutionalization. Since approximately one-half of the elderly are supported by some form of public assistance, the ability to afford nursing home care is not a factor (although it can influence the type of nursing home entered or the ability to purchase community-based care options). Medical problems are less significant to institutionalization than the individual's level of function.

87. A new staff member feels it would be uplifting and invigorating to the residents of the nursing home for the residents to change their rooms and roommates. Your best response to this suggestion is:

a. "There is a risk of more negative than positive outcomes from this type of change."
b. "All of the residents will have some type of physical reaction from this move."
c. "This type of change is known to improve the functional capacity of nursing home residents."
d. "This type of change has been shown to have benefit for residents and staff."

The stress incurred in being moved from one location to another is known as relocation trauma. Although it is most commonly thought to be associated when patients move from the community to an institution or from one institution to another, disrupting the nursing home resident's immediate environment by changing rooms or roommates can be equally stressful. A variety of physical and psychological health threats result from relocation trauma.

To minimize the negative effects of relocation it is important to give the older adult control and choice in the move, and to minimize the unpredictables. For instance, if a relocation of nursing home residents is necessary, it would be useful to discuss the move with residents, have them visit their new rooms, allow them to take personal belongings to the new room, encourage them to express their feelings, and maintain the same routines as in the former location.

Legal Aspects

88. *You receive a call from the son of one of your nursing home residents who tells you that his father is writing letters to family members telling them that the son is "an inconsiderate, greedy liar who is just interested in his inheritance." The son says he is embarrassed by his father's behavior and asks that you take his father's letters from the outgoing mail bin and give them to the son before they can be mailed. Your appropriate action should be:*

a. Follow the son's request
b. Read all the letters before they are mailed and include an explanatory note if the letter is inflammatory
c. Continue to allow the letters to be mailed
d. Refuse to supply writing paper to the resident and ask him to speak with his son about the matter

People do not forfeit their basic rights upon admission to an institution. The Patient's Bill of Rights lists one of the rights of nursing home patients to be to receive and send mail unopened. To invade this resident's rights is to invade his privacy. If the son is concerned with his father's attitude toward him perhaps some counseling with the two could prove useful. You need to inform the son that your responsibility to your patient prevents you from following his request.

89. *Which is not an accurate statement regarding elder abuse?*

    a. It can consist of physical, psychological, financial, or sexual acts.

    b. There are laws protecting the elderly from abuse.

    c. Most abuse is committed by persons close to the older adult.

    d. Older individuals readily report their abuse once they are aware of the reporting procedure.

Many acts constitute abuse, such as theft, inflicting pain or injury, misusing drugs, exploiting, withholding necessities, or threatening to harm. Abuse can occur in any setting, by any person, although most is committed by someone close to the older person—a caregiver, for example. Although laws exist to protect the elderly from abuse, most older individuals are reluctant to report their abuse. They may fear repercussions, embarrassment at admitting to a family member treating them in this fashion, or be concerned that they may be relocated to a less desirable situation (i.e., being abused while living in a son's home may be viewed as less offensive than living in an institution). Gerontological nurses should report all cases of actual or suspected abuse; since reporting mechanisms can very by state, obtain guidance from the local agency on aging.

90. *You are the evening supervisor in a small nursing home. You notice that one of your patients is coughing and has a low-grade fever. You call the physician and say that you believe the patient is developing pneumonia. The physician gives a telephone order for an antibiotic and says he will visit the patient first thing tomorrow. During the night, the patient's condition worsens, and he dies en route to the hospital from what is later determined to be a myocardial infarction. The family brings a lawsuit against you and the physician. In terms of liability:*

a. **You and the physician can be held responsible for malpractice**
b. Only the physician is responsible
c. Only you are responsible
d. Only the facility can be sued

Professional nurses constitute a minority of the nursing staff in long-term care facilities and usually hold positions of great responsibility. With this responsibility comes the added risk of legal problems. As the supervisor in this example, you probably have many problems to manage and tremendous demands by subordinates, patients, and visitors. It is likely that you've seen dozens of patients with pneumonia before, and this particular patient resembles the others. Thus, you conclude that she, too, has pneumonia; this is your first mistake. It is beyond the legal scope of nursing practice to diagnose a medical problem. You should have collected all the data, communicated it to the physician, and held the physician responsible for making the diagnosis. Since you made a medical diagnosis, you failed to abide by the standards for the nursing profession and could be liable for malpractice. Of course, the physician was also negligent in not obtaining and validating appropriate data. You both could be liable.

This question also demonstrates the difficulties resulting from telephone orders. Without patients in front of them, physicians must rely on the data communicated by nurses when telephone orders are obtained. Incomplete or inaccurate sharing of information can result in inappropriate treatment. Physicians may forget all the medications patients are receiving or not be aware of changes in status and order treatments contrary to patients' best interests. Also, orders may be incorrectly stated or heard, such as 25 mg instead of .25 mg. It may not be realistic to eliminate telephone orders, but legal risks can be reduced if nurses:

- collect and communicate a comprehensive database to the physician
- review the medications administered and recent vital signs
- don't diagnose the problem
- obtain the order directly from the physician, not via a secretary or office nurse
- write the order as it is given

- repeat the order to the physician in its entirety
- question inappropriate or unusual orders
- request the physician to visit the patient if there is any doubt or question as to the patient's status
- have the order signed within 24 hours

91. *The physician is concerned that 72-year-old Mrs. J will be upset if the need for her surgery is fully explained to her and consults with Mr. J to obtain consent for surgery. Mr. J tells the physician to obtain consent from their son who "is better able to understand these things." In reference to this consent, you know that:*

    a. Mrs. J must grant consent
    b. Only the next of kin can grant consent, which in this case would be Mr. J
    c. Any blood relative can grant consent if the patient will be disturbed by the explanation of the procedure
    d. The physician should obtain consent from Mrs. J, but omit explaining the procedure and its risks

Consent is required for any procedure that exceeds basic care measures. Unless a patient has been legally judged as incompetent and a guardian appointed to act in his or her behalf, consent must be obtained from the patient. Consent must be informed, that is, the procedure, its purpose, expected results, risks, and alternative options must be explained; consent for research participation must be obtained also. The person performing the procedure should be responsible for explaining the procedure and obtaining consent. The consent form is signed by the patient and the person witnessing the consent (Pozgar 1983, 98-110). The fact that Mrs. J may be upset if she has the surgery explained to her or that her son will be better able to understand the explanation does not eliminate the need to obtain consent from her.

Nurses should assure that patients fully understand the consent they are granting. Medical jargon, the inability to read the small print on the form, and a reluctance to ask questions may cause patients to sign consent forms without fully understanding implications. Clarification and advocacy for patients may be necessary.

Gerontological nurses may find a variety of potential liabilities in their practices. For example, placing a "DNR" on the patient's care plan because the physician mentioned that the patient shouldn't be coded is invalid unless it has been written as a medical order; allowing an employee with whom you're not familiar to work on your unit will not relieve you of liability for his actions under the doctrine of *respondeat superior;* telling a patient that you're going to lock him in a room if he isn't quiet can be viewed as assault; and writing a bad reference on a former employee based on your perceptions rather than on fact can constitute defamation of character. With an increasingly litigious society, it behooves gerontological nurses to be knowledgeable about legal issues and to assure legally sound nursing practice.

Reimbursement

92. *Medicare is a:*

    a. Program of no-cost health insurance for persons age 65 and over, and for the poor of all ages
    b. Contributory health insurance program for persons age 65 and over
    c. Health insurance program for the poor of all ages
    d. Federal health insurance program for persons unable to qualify for private health insurance

In 1965, the Social Security program was expanded to include Medicare (Title 18). Part A of Medicare is free to eligible elderly and covers hospital, home health, and skilled nursing home services with specific limitations. Part B is an optional coverage for physician's services, outpatient therapy, some medical supplies, and unlimited home health visits. The elderly are expected to pay for those services not covered by the program.

Medicaid is a health insurance program for low-income persons of all ages. Elderly persons may qualify for this program after their other benefits have been exhausted and they meet the eligibility requirements. The type of care covered by Medicaid varies from state to state.

93. *Medicare reimburses for:*

    a. Only hospital bills
    b. Hospital and physician bills

    c. Hospital and physician bills and unlimited nursing home care
    d. Medical, surgical, dental, and nursing care in any Medicare participating agency

Although nursing home care may be reimbursed by Medicare, it is not unlimited. Dental care and routine preventive health care measures are not covered by the program, either.

Assuring Quality

94. *Which is a valid statement regarding the regulation of health care practice?*
    a. Local city and county governments do not have the authority to develop regulations.
    b. Federal regulations are optional if state regulations exist.
    c. Agencies who accept only private-pay patients are exempt from regulations.
    d. State regulations can be more stringent than federal regulations.

Federal, state, and local governments can develop standards, survey agencies, and impose sanctions as part of their regulatory process. Regulations exist for various types of health care services, such as skilled nursing homes, home health agencies, and medical day care. For reimbursement purposes, agencies must meet the "conditions of participation," or standards, described in federal law, although there are a variety of additional standards that must be met to maintain licensure of the health care agency. Federal regulations are considered the minimum standards to be met by an agency, and states can include additional requirements in their regulations. Again, regulations are minimum standards; gerontological nurses should try to aspire to higher levels of standards in their practices, such as those developed by the American Nurses' Association, the Joint Commission on the Accreditation of Hospitals (JCAH), and other professional organizations.

95. *Which of the following would you not recognize as part of the ANA Standards for Gerontological Nursing?*

a. Data are systematically and continuously collected about the health status of the older adult.
b. **A plan of nursing care is developed according to the prescribed medical plan.**
c. The plan of nursing care includes priorities and prescribed approaches.
d. The older adult and significant others participate in deter mining progress attained in achieving goals.

Certainly, the medical plan of care is important to know and consider, but it will not direct the plan of nursing care. Nursing care plans are derived from the nursing assessment and nursing diagnoses. Nursing looks at all aspects of the individual and should not be limited to the medical plan.

In addition to emphasizing the importance of the nursing process, the ANA Standards reinforce the necessity for the older adult and significant others to participate in that process.

96. *The basic foundations upon which a strong quality assurance program is built are:*

a. Audits
b. **Standards**
c. Policies and procedures
d. QA plans

Standards are the accepted practices that describe what the practitioner or agency hopes to accomplish, and are the basis for practice. From standards, policies emerge, stating the principles behind actions, and procedures, describing the specific steps in implementing the action. Audits are performed to determine if the standards have been set. Quality assurance plans are important to a strong program, but they require standards on which to be built.

97. *A director of nursing wants to determine if all medications given over the past month have been signed by a licensed nurse at the appropriate times. This type of audit is:*

a. **Structure**
b. Outcome

c. Concurrent
d. Process

Audits are a way to determine if actual practice is consistent with the standards of care, and they can take several forms:

- *structure:* looking at the resources and practices in relation to stated standards without consideration of outcomes
- *process:* reviewing the actual actions being followed and how they match with standards
- *outcome:* examining the final result

Audits can also be described according to the timeframe used for evaluation:

- *retrospective:* past
- *concurrent:* present
- *prospective:* future

The director of nursing in this question wants to examine structures in a retrospective manner.

98. *The staff want to initiate a 15 minute/day exercise program with a select group of elderly to see if there will be any decrease in their arthritis symptoms. To determine if the desired results are being achieved, you would want to conduct which type of audit?*

a. Structure
b. Outcome
c. Retrospective
d. Process

The end results are of interest in this situation; thus, an outcome audit is utilized.

Research

99. *One major problem of past gerontological research has been:*

a. Insufficient studies of institutionalized populations
b. High proportion of replicated studies

c. Too much reliance on conceptual models
d. Poor methodology

Gerontological nursing, along with the field of gerontology in general, has not had a proud past where research is concerned. With an undeveloped specialty and few gerontological nurses prepared to research, studies often lacked theoretical frameworks, conceptual models, and adequate replication. Too many studies focused on the institutionalized elderly who were not representative of the majority of older adults. Since the 1970s, this situation has changed. Well-trained nurse researchers are contributing their impressive analytical skills to the field. The National Institute on Aging has promoted and funded research benefiting gerontological nursing. Continued research is necessary as the evolving specialty of gerontological nursing continues to build its knowledge base and learns effective strategies for caring for the aged.

Gerontological Nursing as a Specialty

100. *Which is an accurate statement about the ANA's Gerontological Nursing Division?*

a. It was one of the earliest specialty divisions.
b. It was officially formed in 1966.
c. It was once part of the American Geriatrics Society.
d. It is considered a subspecialty of the medical-surgical nursing division.

Nursing has long been the backbone of manpower in providing services to older adults, but it was not until 1961 that the ANA recommended forming a specialty group for geriatric nurses. This group met in 1962 for the first time as the Conference Group on Geriatric Nursing Practice. In 1966, the Division of Geriatric Nursing Practice was officially launched within the ANA. The name was changed 10 years later to the Gerontological Nursing Division to reflect the nursing role with all aging persons, not just the ill aged. The specialty has grown tremendously since that time, increasing its knowledge base, literature, and professional pool. As the numbers and needs of the older population continue to grow, so will the demand for additional, competent gerontological nurses.

References

Burnside, I.M. 1984. *Working with the elderly: Group process and techniques. 2d ed.* Monterey, CA: Wadsworth.

Butler, R.N., and M.I. Lewis. 1982. *Aging and mental health.* St. Louis: C.V. Mosby Co., 58-59.

Cumming, E., and W.E. Henry. 1961. *Growing old: The process of disengagement.* New York: Basic Books.

Ebersole, P. 1976. Problems of group reminiscing with the institutionalized aged. *Journal of Gerontological Nursing* 2(6):23-27.

Erikson, E. 1963. *Childhood and society. 2d ed.* New York: WW Norton.

Few, A., and R. Getty. 1967. Occurrence of lipofuscin as related to aging in the canine and porcine nervous system. *Journal of Gerontology* 22:357-367.

Havighurst, R.J. 1963. Successful aging. In *Processes of aging,* Williams, R.H., C. Tibbitts, and W. Donahue, edited by Williams, R.H. Vol I, 299-320. New York, Atherton Press.

Johnson, C.L., and L.A. Grant. 1985. *The nursing home in American society.* Baltimore: Johns Hopkins University Press.

Knudsen, F.S. 1984. Cardiovascular conditions in older adults. In *Handbook of gerontological nursing,* edited by Steffl, B.M. New York: Van Nostrand Reinhold Co., Inc.

National Center for Health Statistics. 1986. Vital statistics of the United States (annual). In U.S. Bureau of the Census, *Statistical abstract of the United States: 1985, 105th ed.,* No. 102.

Neugarten, B.L. 1964. *Personality in middle and late life.* New York: Atherton Press.

Peck, R.C. 1956. Psychological development in the second half of late life. In *Psychological Aspects of Aging,* edited by Anderson, J.E. Washington, DC: American Psychological Association.

Pozgar, G.D. 1983. *Legal aspects of health care administration. 2d ed.* Rockville, MD: Aspen Systems Corp.

U.S. Bureau of the Census. 1986a. *Statistical abstract of the United States: 1985, 105th ed.,* No. 102, p.69.

U.S. Bureau of the Census. 1986b. *Current population reports,* series P-60, No. 144.

U.S. Bureau of the Census. 1986c. *Statistical abstract of the United States: 105th ed.,* No. 178, p.111.

Selected Bibliography

Facts About The Older Population

Demographics

Brock, A.M. 1984. From wife to widowhood: A changing life-style. *Journal of Gerontological Nursing* 10(4):8-15.

Brody, E.M. 1985. Parent care as a normative stress. *Gerontologist* 25(1):19-29.

Fillenbaum, G.G. 1984. Change in the household composition of the elderly: A preliminary investigation. *Journal of Gerontology* 39(3):342-349.

Mitchell, J. 1984. An exploration of family interaction with the elderly by race, socioeconomic status, and residence. *Gerontologist* 24(1):48-54.

Rosenwaike, I., and B. Logue. 1985. *The extreme aged in America: A portrait of an expanding population.* Westport, CT: Greenwood Press, Inc.

U.S. Bureau of the Census. 1985. *Current Population Reports.* Washington, DC: Government Printing Office.

Cultural Aspects

Branch, M.F., and P.P. Paxton, eds. 1976. *Providing safe nursing care for ethnic people of color.* New York: Appleton-Century-Crofts.

Clavon, A.M., and V.P. Smith. 1986. One black couple's means of coping: preserving identity. *Journal of Gerontological Nursing.* 12(1):26-28.

Dibner, A.S. 1982. Ethnic and cultural variations in the care of the aged. *Journal of Geriatric Psychiatry.* 15(2):193-196.

Fry, C.L., ed. 1980. *Aging in culture and society: Comparative viewpoints and strategies.* Brooklyn: J.F. Bergin Publishers.

Kalish R.A., and Moriwaki, S. 1979. The world of the elderly Asian American. In *Dimensions of aging: Readings,* edited by Hendricks, J., and C.D. Hendricks, 264-277. Cambridge, MA: Winthrop Publishers.

Manuel, R.C., ed. 1982. *Minority aging: Sociological and social psychological issues.* Westport, CT: Greenwood Press.

Mitchell, J. 1984. An exploration of family interaction with the elderly by race, socioeconomic status, and residence. *Gerontologist* 24(1):48-54.

Financial Aspects

Champlin, L. 1983. Early retirement: A catalyst for health problems? *Geriatrics* 38(7):106-109.

Streib, G.F. 1983. Two views of retirement: In the clinic and in the community. In *Clinical aspects of aging,* edited by Reichel, W., 533-539. 2d ed. Baltimore: Williams and Wilkens.

Rates of Illness

U.S. National Center for Health Statistics. *Vital statistics of the U.S.* Washington, DC: Government Printing Office.

Theories Of Aging

Biological Aging

Blumenthal, H.T. 1983. Biology of aging. In *Care of the geriatric patient,* edited by Steinburg, F.U., 18-38. 6th ed. St. Louis: C.V. Mosby Co.

Goldman, R. 1984. Normal human aging: A theoretical context. In *Geriatric medicine,* edited by Cassel, C.K., and J.R. Walsh, Vol. I, 3-12. New York: Springer-Verlag.

Meier, D.E. 1984. The cell biology of aging. In *Geriatric medicine,* edited by Cassel, C.K., and J.R. Walsh, Vol. I, 3-12. New York: Springer-Verlag.

Steinburg, F.U. 1983. The aging of organs and organ systems. In *Care of the geriatric patient,* edited by Steinburg, F.U., 3-17. 6th ed., St. Louis: C.V. Mosby Co.

Psychological Aging

Atchley, R.D. 1983. *Aging, continuity, and change.* Belmont, CA: Wadsworth Press.

Baltes, P., and S.L. Willis. 1977. Toward psychological theories of aging and development. In *Handbook of the psychology of aging,* edited by Birren, J.E. and W. Schaie, 128-154. New York: Van Nostrand Reinhold Co.

Erikson, E. 1963. *Childhood and society.* 2d ed. New York: W.W. Norton.

Kimmel, D.C. 1980. *Adulthood and aging.* 2d ed. New York: Wiley.

Peck, R.C. 1956. Psychological developments in the second half of late life. In *Psychological aspects of aging,* edited by Anderson, J.E. Washington, D.C.: American Psychological Association.

Physical Aging And Nursing Response
Cardiovascular Changes

deVries, H.H. 1984. Exercise. In *Geriatric medicine,* edited by Cassel, C.K., and J.R. Walsh, Vol. II, 175-177. New York: Springer-Verlag.

Downey, K.K., and B.K. Davis. 1986. Measuring blood pressure via sensory detection. *Journal of Gerontological Nursing.* 12(11):8-11.

Hitzhusen, J.C. 1984. The elderly heart: Special signs and symptoms to watch for. *Geriatrics* 39(6):38-51.

Orem, S.E. 1984. Assessment of the cardiovascular system. In *Health assessment of the older adult,* edited by Eliopoulos, C., 81-97. Menlo Park, CA: Addison-Wesley Publishing Co.

Respiratory Changes

Acee, S. 1984. Helping patients breathe more easily... non-invasive nursing measures. *Geriatric Nursing* 5(6):230-233.

Sigmon, H.D. 1984. Assessment of the respiratory system. In *Health assessment of the older adult,* edited by Eliopoulos, C., 81-97. Menlo Park, CA: Addison-Wesley Publishing Co.

Gastrointestinal Changes

Eliopoulos, C. 1984. Assessment of the gastrointestinal system. In *Health assessment of the older adult,* edited by Eliopoulos, C., 99-124. Menlo Park, CA: Addison-Wesley Publishing Co.

Hudis, M.M. 1983. Dentistry for the elderly. In *Clinical aspects of aging,* edited by Reichel, W., 198-509. 2d ed. Baltimore: Williams and Wilkens.

Genitourinary Changes

Breschi, L. 1983. Common lower urinary tract problems in the elderly. In *Clinical aspects of aging,* edited by Reichel, W., 302-318. 2d. ed. Baltimore: Williams and Wilkens.

Eliopoulos, C. 1984. Assessment of the urinary system. In *Health assessment of the older adult,* edited by Eliopoulos, C., 179-188. Menlo Park, CA: Addison-Wesley Publishing Co.

Jessup, L.E. 1984. The chest, abdomen, and genitourinary system. In *Handbook of gerontological nursing,* edited by Steffl, B.M., 193-206. New York: Van Nostrand Reinhold Co.

Masters, W.H., and V. Johnson. 1981. Sex and the aging process. *Journal of the American Geriatrics Society* 29(9):385-390.

McConnell, J. 1984. Preventing urinary tract infections. *Geriatric Nursing* 5(8):361-362.

Steinke, E.E., and M.B. Bergen. 1986. Sexuality and aging. *Journal of Gerontological Nursing* 12(6):6-10.

Sensory Changes

Kasper, R.L. 1983. Eye problems in the aged. In *Clinical aspects of aging,* edited by Reichel, W., 479-488. 2d. ed. Baltimore: Williams and Wilkens.

Meyd, C.J. 1984. Assessment of the nervous system. In *Health assessment of the older adult,* edited by Eliopoulos, C., 145-168. Menlo Park, CA: Addison-Wesley Publishing Co.

Rose, M.A. 1986. Sensory loss simulation use in nursing education. *Journal of Gerontological Nursing* 12(7):22-24.

Steffl, B.M. 1984. Sensory deprivation in the elderly. In *Handbook of gerontological nursing,* edited by Steffl, B.M., 50-66. New York: Van Nostrand Reinhold Co.

Weinstock, F.J. 1983. When to refer to an opthalmologist. *Geriatrics* 38(11):117-124.

Body Temperature

Higgins, P. 1983. Can 98.6 be a fever in disguise? *Geriatric Nursing* 4(2):101-104.

Kolanowski, A., and L. Gunther. 1981. Hypothermia in the elderly. *Geriatric Nursing* 2(5):362-365.

Skin Changes

Berliner, H. 1986. Aging skin. *American Journal of Nursing.* Part I, 86(10):1138-1141; Part II, 86(11):1259-1261.

Shelley, W.B. and E.D. Shelley. 1982. The ten major problems of aging skin. *Geriatrics* 37(10):107.

Sleep

Bahr, R.T. 1983. Sleep-wake patterns in the aged. *Journal of Gerontological Nursing* 9(10):534-537, 549-541.

Spiegel, R. 1981. *Sleep and sleeplessness in advanced age.* New York: S.P. Medical and Scientific Books.

Diet

Beattie, B.L., and V.Y. Louie. 1983. Nutrition and health in the elderly. In *Clinical aspects of aging,* edited by Reichel, W., 248-270. Baltimore: Williams and Wilkens.

Cadigan, M. 1984. Nutrition and the elderly. In *Handbook of gerontological nursing,* edited by Steffl, B.M., 377-393. New York: Van Nostrand Reinhold Co.

Drugay, M. 1986. Nutritional evaluation: Who needs it? *Journal of Gerontological Nursing* 12(4):14-18.

Masaro, E.J. 1985. Nutrition and aging—a current assessment. *Journal of nutrition* 115(7):842-848.

Natow, A.B. 1980. *Geriatric nutrition.* Boston: CBI Publishing Co.

Yen, P. 1984. Assessment of nutritional status. In *Health assessment of the older adult,* edited by Eliopoulos, C., 125-144. Menlo Park, CA: Addison-Wesley Publishing Co.

Health Problems And Nursing Response

Cardiovascular Problems

Coyle, J.F., and L.L. Basta. 1983. Unstable angina pectoris. *Geriatrics.* 38(9):79-92.

Deckert, J., and R. Hom. 1983. Cardiovascular disease in the elderly: Diagnostic dilemma. *Geriatrics* 38(2):48-52.

Hitzhusen, J.C. 1984. The elderly heart: Special signs and symptoms to watch for. *Geriatrics* 39(6):38-51.

Knudsen, F.S. 1984. Cardiovascular conditions in older adults. In *Handbook of gerontological nursing,* edited by Steffl, B.M., 221-233. New York: Van Nostrand Reinhold Co.

McDonald, W.J. 1984. Hypertension. In *Geriatric medicine,* edited by Cassel, C.K. and J.R. Walsh, Vol. I, 183-196. New York: Springer-Verlag.

Spittell, J.A. 1983. Diagnosis and management of leg ulcer. *Geriatrics.* 38(6):57-68.

Webb, C.L. 1984. Sudden cardiac death: An approach to management. *Geriatrics.* 39(4):49-61.

Zoler, M.L. 1984. MI: Recent insights and new treatments? *Geriatrics* 39(5):123-136.

Respiratory Problems

Acee, S. 1984. Helping patients breathe more easily. *Geriatric nursing* 5(6):230-233.

Morris, J.F. 1984. Pulmonary diseases. In *Geriatric medicine,* edited by Cassel, C.K. and J.R. Walsh, Vol. I, 122-146. New York: Springer-Verlag.

Mostow, S.R. 1983. Infectious complications in the elderly COPD patient. *Geriatrics* 38(10):42-49.

Gastrointestinal Problems

Davis, A., et al. 1986. Bowel management. A quality assurance approach to upgrading programs. *Journal of Gerontological Nursing* 12(5):13-18.

Eastwood, G.L. 1984. GI problems in the elderly. *Geriatrics* 39(5):59-86

Knudsen, F.S. 1984. Gastrointestinal and metabollic problems in older adults. In *Handbook of gerontological nursing,* edited by Steffl, B.M., 234-250. New York: Van Nostrand Reinhold.

Kravitz, S.C. 1983. Anemia in the elderly. In *Clinical aspects of aging,* edited by Reichel, W., 443-452. 2d ed. Baltimore: Williams and Wilkens.

Yatto, R.P. 1984. Cholestasis: An alternative to surgery in older patients. *Geriatrics* 39(5):113-122.

Diabetes

Bennett, P.H. 1984. Diabetes in the elderly: Diagnosis and epidemiology. *Geriatrics* 39(5):36-44.

Istre, S. 1984. Daily and monthly diabetic flowsheets. *Geriatric nursing* 5(8):363-365.

Levin, M.E. 1983. Diabetes mellitus. In *Care of the geriatric patient,* edited by Steinburg, F.U., 154-181. 6th ed. St. Louis: C.V. Mosby Co.

Genitourinary Problems

Frentz, G.D., and D.P. Bell. 1983. Managing urinary tract infections in the geriatric population. *Geriatrics* 38(11):42-50.

Greengold, B.A., and J.G. Ouslander. 1986. Bladder retraining. *Journal of Gerontological Nursing.* 12(6):31-35.

Lindner, A., P. Jonas, and A. Ohrv. 1983. Postprostactectomy impotence in elderly patients. *Geriatrics* 38(9):113-117.

Kendall, A.R., and B.S. Stein. 1983. Stress urinary incontinence. *Geriatrics* 38(5):69-79.

Ruge, C.A. 1986. Shock (wave) treatment for kidney stones. *American Journal of Nursing* 86(4):400-402.

Neurological Problems

Eifrig, D.E., and K.B. Simons. 1983. An overview of common geriatric opthalmologic disorders. *Geriatrics* 38(4):55-79.

Fisher, M.A. 1984. Peripheral neuropathies: A common complaint in older patients. *Geriatrics* 39(2):115-129.

Hart, G. 1983. Strokes causing left versus right hemiplegia: Different effects and nursing implications. *Geriatric nursing* 4(1):39-43.

Rappaport, B.Z. 1984. Audiology. In *Geriatric medicine,* edited by Cassel, C.K., and J.R. Walsh, Vol. I, 111-121. New York: Springer-Verlag.

Musculoskeletal Problems

Albert, S.F., and D.W. Jahnigan. 1983. Common foot disorders among the elderly. *Geriatrics* 38(6):42-55.

Avioloi, L.V. 1983. Aging, bone, and osteoporosis. In *Care of the geriatric patient,* edited by Steinburg, F.U., 143-153. 6th ed. St. Louis: C.V. Mosby Co.

Lane, J.M., V.J. Vigorita, and M. Falls. 1984. Osteoporosis: Current diagnosis and treatment. *Geriatrics* 39(4):40-48.

Lukens, L. 1986. Six months after hip fracture. *Geriatric nursing* 7(4):202-206.

Moskowitz, R.W. 1983. Arthritis in the elderly: Some observations. *Geriatrics* 39(10):66-78.

Mental Health And Illness

Assessment

Antoine, M., C. Holland, and B. Scruggs. 1986. Measuring improvement in patients with dementia. *Geriatric nursing.* 7(4):185-189.

Brody, E. 1984. *Mental and physical health practices of older people.* New York: Springer Publishing Co.

Lucas, M.J. 1984. Assessment of mental status. In *Health assessment of the older adult,* edited by Eliopoulos, C., 169-176. Menlo Park, CA: Addison-Wesley Publishing Co.

Lucas, M.J., C. Steele, and A. Bognanni. 1986. Recognition of psychiatric symptoms in dementia. *Journal of Gerontological Nursing* 12(1):11-15.

Wolanin, M.O., and L.R.P. Phillips. 1981. *Confusion: Prevention and care.* St. Louis: C.V. Mosby Co.

Depression

Blazer, D.G. 1982. *Depression in late life.* St. Louis: C.V. Mosby Co.

Burnside, I.M. 1984. Life crisis reactions, depression, and paranoia. In *Handbook of gerontological nursing,* edited by Steffl, B.M., 97-106. New York: Van Nostrand Reinhold.

Chaisson-Stewart, G.M., ed. 1985. *Depression in the elderly: An interdisciplinary approach.* New York: John Wiley and Sons, Inc.

Gaitz, C.M. 1983. Indentifying and treating depression in an older patient. *Geriatrics* 38(2):42-46.

Hall, R.C.W. 1984. Tricyclic antidepressants in the treatment of the elderly. *Geriatrics* 39(4):81-95.

Harris, M. 1986. Helping the person with an altered self-image. *Geriatric Nursing* 7(2):90-93.

Dementia

Akerlund, B.M., and A. Norberg. 1986. Group psychotherapy with demented patients. *Geriatric Nursing* 7(2):83-84.

American College of Physician's Report. 1983. Toward an effective treatment of Alzheimer's disease. *Annals of Internal Medicine* 98:251.

Clites, J. 1984. Maximizing memory retention in the aged. *Journal of Gerontological Nursing* 10(8):34-35, 38-39.

Francis, G., and A. Baly. 1986. Plush animals—Do they make a difference? *Geriatric Nursing* 7(3):140-142.

Gaffney, J. 1986. Toward a less restrictive environment. *Geriatric Nursing* 7(2):94-96.

Hall, G., M.V. Kirschling, and S. Todd. 1986. Sheltered freedom: An Alzheimer's unit in an ICF. *Geriatric nursing* 7(3):132-137.

Rabins, P.V., and M.F. Folstein. 1983. The demented patient: Evaluation and care. *Geriatrics* 38(8):99-106.

Schafer, S.C. 1985. Modifying the environment for patients with Alzheimer's disease. *Geriatric Nursing* 6(3):157-159.

Grief

Albert, M.V.L., and B.M. Steffl. 1984. Loss, grief, and death in old age. In *Handbook of gerontological nursing,* edited by Steffl, B.M., 73-87. New York: Van Nostrand Reinhold Co.

Lund, D.A. 1984. Can pets help the bereaved? *Journal of Gerontological Nursing* 10(6):8-12.

Geropharmacology

Albrick, J.M. 1984. Geriatric pharmacology. In *Geriatric emergencies,* edited by Schwartz, G.R., G. Bosker, and J.W. Grigsley, 84-106. Bowie, MD: Robert J. Brady Co.

Berlinger, W.G. 1984. Adverse drug reactions in the elderly. *Geriatrics* 39(5):45-58.

Jerigan, J.A. 1984. Update on drugs and the elderly. *American Family Physician* 29(4):238-247.

Keenan, R., et al. 1983. The benefits of a drug holiday. *Geriatric Nursing* 4(2):103-104.

Lamy, P.P. 1986. Drug interactions and the elderly. *Journal of Gerontological Nursing* 12(2):36-37.

Lamy, P.P. 1984. Use of hypnotics in the elderly. *American Family Physician* 30(2):187-191.

Oppeneer, J.E., and T.M. Vervoren. 1983. *Gerontological pharmacology. A resource book for health practitioners.* St. Louis: C.V. Mosby Co.

Pagliaro, L.A., and A.M. Pagliaro. 1986. Age-dependent drug selection and response. In *Pharmacologic aspects of nursing,* edited by Pagliaro, A.M., and L.A. Pagliaro. St. Louis: C.V. Mosby Co.

Pagliaro, L.A., and A.M. Pagliaro, eds. 1983. *Pharmacologic aspects of aging.* St. Louis: C.V. Mosby Co.

Todd, B. 1986. Transdermal nitroglycerin ointment and patches. *Geriatric Nursing* 7(3):152.

Practice Issues

Service Delivery

Brody, S.J., and N.A. Persily. 1984. *Hospitals and the aged. The new old market.* Rockville, MD: Aspen Systems Corp.

Eliopoulos, C. 1983. *Nursing administration of long term care.* Rockville, MD: Aspen Systems Corp.

Fox, N. 1986. *You, your parent, and the nursing home: The family's guide to long-term care.* Buffalo, NY: Prometheus Books.

Friedman, J. 1986. *Home health care: A complete guide for patients and their families.* New York, W.W. Norton and Co.

Gallagher, A.P. 1986. A model for change in long term care. *Journal of Gerontological Nursing* 12(5):19-23.

Hall, J.E., and B.R. Weaver, eds. 1985. *Distributive nursing practice. A systems approach to community health.* Philadelphia: J.B. Lippincott Co.

Johnson, C.L., and L.A. Grant. 1985. *The nursing home in American society.* Baltimore: Johns Hopkins University Press.

Killeffer, E.H.P., R. Bennett, and G. Gruen. 1985. *Handbook of innovative programs for the impaired elderly.* New York: Haworth Press.

O'Brien, C.L. 1982. *Adult day care: A practical guide.* Monterey, CA: Wadsworth Health Sciences Division.

Somers, A. 1985. Preventive health services for the elderly. In *Principles of geriatric medicine,* edited by Andres, R. New York: McGraw Hill Book Co.

Legal Aspects

Beck, C.M., and L.R. Phillips. 1982. Abuse of the elderly. *Journal of Gerontological Nursing* 8(2):22-26.

Fox, T.C., ed. 1986. *Long-term care and the law.* Owings Mills, MD: Rynd Communications.

Henry, K.H. 1984. *The health care supervisor's legal guide.* Rockville, MD: Aspen Systems Corp.

Reimbursement

Baines, E. 1984. Medicare and medicaid—differences and similarities. *Journal of Gerontological Nursing* 10(1):36-37.

Davis, K., and D. Rowland. 1986. *Medicare policy. New directions for health and long term care.* Baltimore: Johns Hopkins University Press.

Assuring Quality

American Nurses' Association. 1985. *Code for nurses with interpretive statements.* Kansas City, MO: American Nurses' Association.

Bandman, E.L., and B. Bandman. 1985. *Nursing ethics in the life span.* Norwalk, CT: Appleton-Century-Crofts.

Hogstel, M.O., ed. 1983. *Management of personnel in long term care.* Bowie, MD: Robert J. Brady Co.

National Health Publishing. 1984. *Operating standards for health care facilities.* Owings Mills, MD: Rynd Communications.

Research

Cora, V.L., and E.D. Lapierre. 1986. ANA speaks out. *Journal of Gerontological Nursing* 12(6):21-26.

Davis, A. 1981. Ethical considerations in gerontological nursing research. *Geriatric Nursing* 2:269.

Thompson, L.F. and B.M. Steffl. 1984. Research in gerontological nursing. In *Handbook of gerontological nursing,* edited by Steffl, B.M., 513-528. New York: Van Nostrand Reinhold Co.

Gerontological Nursing as a Specialty

American Nurses' Association. 1976. *Standards of gerontological nursing practice.* Kansas City, MO: American Nurses' Association.

American Nurses' Association. 1983. *Take the extra step: Become a certified nurse.* Kansas City, MO: American Nurses' Association.

Brock, A. 1984. Gerontological nursing in the 80's: Fight or flight? *Journal of Gerontological Nursing* 10(3):102.

Davis, B.A. 1983. The gerontological nursing specialty. *Journal of Gerontological Nursing* 9(10):526-532.

Division on Gerontological Nursing Practice. 1981. *A statement on the scope of gerontological nursing practice.* Kansas City, MO: American Nurses' Association.

Schwab, M. 1983. Professional nursing and the care of the aged. In *Clinical aspects of aging,* edited by Reichel, W., 564-569. 2d ed. Baltimore: Williams and Wilkens.

Wells, D.L. 1985. Gerontological nurse specialists: Tomorrow's leaders today! Role implementation strategies. *Journal of Gerontological Nursing* 11(5):36-40.

Annotated Bibliography

American Nurses' Association. 1976. *Standards of gerontological nursing practice*. Kansas City, MO: American Nurses' Association.

Standards form the foundation for practice, and in this short publication, the ANA describes the general framework for gerontological nursing practice.

Burnside, I.M., ed. 1981. *Nursing and the aged*. 2d ed. New York: McGraw-Hill Book Co.

This comprehensive text is particularly strong in its discussion of normal aging and psychosocial aspects of nursing older adults. Chapters are contributed by many expert leaders in various disciplines.

Carnevali, D.L., and M. Patrick, eds. 1986. *Nursing management for the elderly*. Philadelphia: J.B. Lippincott Co.

This well-organized book combines theory with practical guidance for delivering services to the elderly. Includes brief summaries of health problems for quick review.

Ebersole, P., and P. Hess. 1985. *Toward healthy aging: Human needs and nursing response*. 2d ed. St. Louis: C.V. Mosby Co.

Using the framework of Maslow's hierarchy of needs, nursing interventions with the elderly are discussed. Strong theoretical explanations are offered as the roles and functions of the geriatric nurse are reviewed.

Eliopoulos, C. 1987. *Gerontological Nursing*. 2d ed. Philadelphia: J.B. Lippincott Co.

A basic, comprehensive text discussing nursing needs of the

healthy and ill elderly. Includes chapters on ethics, legal issues, service delivery, and other issues relevant to the practicing nurse.

Ham, R.J., ed. 1986. *Geriatric medicine annual.* New Jersey: Medical Economics Books.

The year 1986 marked the introduction of this annual publication that will share the most recent advances and changes in the field of geriatric medicine. In this rapidly growing specialty, this book is a useful resource in staying current.

Kane, R., and R. Kane. 1981. *Assessing the elderly: A practical guide to measurement.* Lexington, MA: Lexington Books.

Discusses the strengths and weaknesses of the various assessment tools and approaches developed for use with the older population.

Murray, R., M. Huelskoetter, and D. O'Driscoll. 1980. *The nursing process in later maturity.* Englewood Cliffs, NJ: Prentice Hall, Inc.

Comprehensive text offering a good balance of theory and practical nursing interventions. Includes objectives for each chapter to guide the reader.

Reichel, W., ed. 1983. *Clinical aspects of aging.* 2d ed. Baltimore: Williams and Wilkens.

Although this is a geriatric medical text, this book provides a good review of the many geriatric health problems nurses confront in practice.

Stilwell, E., ed. 1980. *Readings in gerontological nursing.* Thorofare, NJ: Charles B. Slack.

This selection of articles from the *Journal of Gerontological Nursing* covers a wide range of issues relevant to gerontological nurses.

Wolanin, M.O., and L. Phillips. 1981. *Confusion: Prevention and care.* St. Louis: C.V. Mosby Co.

This book provides an indepth study of the many causes of mental health problems and related nursing assessment techniques and interventions.

Hints for Taking the Test

Many nurses, particularly those who have not been in school for a while, panic when faced with a multiple-choice examination. Often, they know the information, but draw a blank when the test booklet is placed before them. Like any other skill, test-taking becomes easier with practice. Nurses planning to take the ANA Certification Exam may find it beneficial to take the test in this book several times, just to get the feel of test-taking and to minimize any anxieties. The following tips should prove useful:

- Arrange your schedule so that you can have approximately two hours of uninterrupted time. You probably won't need all that time, but it is far better to overestimate your time requirements than to work under pressure to finish within an underestimated deadline.

- Find a quiet area that has a desk and chair. If you're planning to sit for the Certification Exam, it is particularly useful to master the discipline of sitting on a hard chair for a block of time, without access to treats or cigarettes!

- Have pen or pencils and some scrap paper available.

- Write down the time you begin so that you will be able to determine with accuracy how much time you really need to complete the exam.

- Tear one of the answer sheets from the text. You may want to duplicate some copies ahead of time so that you'll have some extras and will not have to damage your book.

- Read each question carefully. Look for the significant points within the question. (Very rarely are facts given that aren't relevant to the answer, so pay attention to every detail).

- Read every answer option. Even if the first answer seems 100 percent correct to you, read them all.

- Pay attention to words such as *not, except, least likely,* and *all but.*
- Look for the *best* answer.
- If you get stumped on a question, move on. Make a note of which question it was on your scrap paper and go back to it when you complete the entire exam. If you still cannot determine the correct answer, choose your best guess.

ANSWER SHEET

1.	a	b	c	d		41.	a	b	c	d
2.	a	b	c	d		42.	a	b	c	d
3.	a	b	c	d		43.	a	b	c	d
4.	a	b	c	d		44.	a	b	c	d
5.	a	b	c	d		45.	a	b	c	d
6.	a	b	c	d		46.	a	b	c	d
7.	a	b	c	d		47.	a	b	c	d
8.	a	b	c	d		48.	a	b	c	d
9.	a	b	c	d		49.	a	b	c	d
10.	a	b	c	d		50.	a	b	c	d
11.	a	b	c	d		51.	a	b	c	d
12.	a	b	c	d		52.	a	b	c	d
13.	a	b	c	d		53.	a	b	c	d
14.	a	b	c	d		54.	a	b	c	d
15.	a	b	c	d		55.	a	b	c	d
16.	a	b	c	d		56.	a	b	c	d
17.	a	b	c	d		57.	a	b	c	d
18.	a	b	c	d		58.	a	b	c	d
19.	a	b	c	d		59.	a	b	c	d
20.	a	b	c	d		60.	a	b	c	d
21.	a	b	c	d		61.	a	b	c	d
22.	a	b	c	d		62.	a	b	c	d
23.	a	b	c	d		63.	a	b	c	d
24.	a	b	c	d		64.	a	b	c	d
25.	a	b	c	d		65.	a	b	c	d
26.	a	b	c	d		66.	a	b	c	d
27.	a	b	c	d		67.	a	b	c	d
28.	a	b	c	d		68.	a	b	c	d
29.	a	b	c	d		69.	a	b	c	d
30.	a	b	c	d		70.	a	b	c	d
31.	a	b	c	d		71.	a	b	c	d
32.	a	b	c	d		72.	a	b	c	d
33.	a	b	c	d		73.	a	b	c	d
34.	a	b	c	d		74.	a	b	c	d
35.	a	b	c	d		75.	a	b	c	d
36.	a	b	c	d		76.	a	b	c	d
37.	a	b	c	d		77.	a	b	c	d
38.	a	b	c	d		78.	a	b	c	d
39.	a	b	c	d		79.	a	b	c	d
40.	a	b	c	d		80.	a	b	c	d

81.	a	b	c	d	91.	a	b	c	d
82.	a	b	c	d	92.	a	b	c	d
83.	a	b	c	d	93.	a	b	c	d
84.	a	b	c	d	94.	a	b	c	d
85.	a	b	c	d	95.	a	b	c	d
86.	a	b	c	d	96.	a	b	c	d
87.	a	b	c	d	97.	a	b	c	d
88.	a	b	c	d	98.	a	b	c	d
89.	a	b	c	d	99.	a	b	c	d
90.	a	b	c	d	100.	a	b	c	d

ANSWER SHEET

1.	a	b	c	d	41.	a	b	c	d
2.	a	b	c	d	42.	a	b	c	d
3.	a	b	c	d	43.	a	b	c	d
4.	a	b	c	d	44.	a	b	c	d
5.	a	b	c	d	45.	a	b	c	d
6.	a	b	c	d	46.	a	b	c	d
7.	a	b	c	d	47.	a	b	c	d
8.	a	b	c	d	48.	a	b	c	d
9.	a	b	c	d	49.	a	b	c	d
10.	a	b	c	d	50.	a	b	c	d
11.	a	b	c	d	51.	a	b	c	d
12.	a	b	c	d	52.	a	b	c	d
13.	a	b	c	d	53.	a	b	c	d
14.	a	b	c	d	54.	a	b	c	d
15.	a	b	c	d	55.	a	b	c	d
16.	a	b	c	d	56.	a	b	c	d
17.	a	b	c	d	57.	a	b	c	d
18.	a	b	c	d	58.	a	b	c	d
19.	a	b	c	d	59.	a	b	c	d
20.	a	b	c	d	60.	a	b	c	d
21.	a	b	c	d	61.	a	b	c	d
22.	a	b	c	d	62.	a	b	c	d
23.	a	b	c	d	63.	a	b	c	d
24.	a	b	c	d	64.	a	b	c	d
25.	a	b	c	d	65.	a	b	c	d
26.	a	b	c	d	66.	a	b	c	d
27.	a	b	c	d	67.	a	b	c	d
28.	a	b	c	d	68.	a	b	c	d
29.	a	b	c	d	69.	a	b	c	d
30.	a	b	c	d	70.	a	b	c	d
31.	a	b	c	d	71.	a	b	c	d
32.	a	b	c	d	72.	a	b	c	d
33.	a	b	c	d	73.	a	b	c	d
34.	a	b	c	d	74.	a	b	c	d
35.	a	b	c	d	75.	a	b	c	d
36.	a	b	c	d	76.	a	b	c	d
37.	a	b	c	d	77.	a	b	c	d
38.	a	b	c	d	78.	a	b	c	d
39.	a	b	c	d	79.	a	b	c	d
40.	a	b	c	d	80.	a	b	c	d

81.	a	b	c	d	91.	a	b	c	d
82.	a	b	c	d	92.	a	b	c	d
83.	a	b	c	d	93.	a	b	c	d
84.	a	b	c	d	94.	a	b	c	d
85.	a	b	c	d	95.	a	b	c	d
86.	a	b	c	d	96.	a	b	c	d
87.	a	b	c	d	97.	a	b	c	d
88.	a	b	c	d	98.	a	b	c	d
89.	a	b	c	d	99.	a	b	c	d
90.	a	b	c	d	100.	a	b	c	d

INDEX

Oxygen, 58-59
Pain
  digitalis toxicity, 78
  glaucoma, 51, 66
  myocardial infarction, 57
Parkinson's disease, 81
Patient's Bill of Rights, 86
Pets, 75-76
Pharmacology, 76-81
Pneumonia, 45-46
  lipoid, 79
Postural drainage, 60
Presbycusis, 52-53
Probenecid, 80-81
Programs for the aged, 30-31
  See also Medicaid, Medicare
Prostatic hypertrophy, 64
Psychotropics, 81
Rectal examination, 61-62
Regulations, health care, 90
Respiratory system, 37, 45-56,
  59-61
Retirement, 41-42
Sexual activity, 49-50, 64-66
Sinusitis, 37
Skin, 54
Social Security, 35, 83, 89
Standards, American Nursing
  Associations for
  Gerontological Nursing,
  56, 90-91
Stress
  Alzheimer's victims, 73
  dementia "catastrophic
    reaction," 72
  glucose intolerance, 63
  mental change, 70
  relocation trauma, 85

  tachycardia, 43
Suicide, 72
Tachycardia, 43
Transient Ischemic Attack
  (TIA), 67
Tardive dyskinesia, 81
Temperature, body, 53-54
  hypothermia, 56
  rheumatoid arthritis symptom,
    67
Theories of aging
  biological, 38-39
  psychological, 38-50
  activity, 40
  developmental or
    continuity, 40-42
  disengagement, 39
Therapy
  antipsychotic or tranquilizer,
    81
  cane use, 68-69
  fracture, 68
  grief, 75
  pet, 75
  pharmaceutical, 76-77
  physical, 43-44
  reminiscence or life review,
    41
Tranquilizers, 81
Transient ischemic attack (TIA),
  66-67
Tuberculosis, 59
Ulcer, stasis, 58
Urine
  See Genitourinary system
Vaginitis, 65
Valsalva maneuver, 58
Varicose veins, 37